Dzhumaboy Rakhmatovich Sanginov
Ilkhomidin Karimovich Niyazov

Reconstructive surgeries in head and neck organ cancer

Dzhumaboy Rakhmatovich Sanginov
Ilkhomidin Karimovich Niyazov

Reconstructive surgeries in head and neck organ cancer

Treatment of head and neck cancer taking into account the quality of life of patients

Imprint

Any brand names and product names mentioned in this book are subject to trademark, brand or patent protection and are trademarks or registered trademarks of their respective holders. The use of brand names, product names, common names, trade names, product descriptions etc. even without a particular marking in this work is in no way to be construed to mean that such names may be regarded as unrestricted in respect of trademark and brand protection legislation and could thus be used by anyone.

Cover image: www.ingimage.com

This book is a translation from the original published under ISBN 978-620-7-45457-0.

Publisher:
Sciencia Scripts
is a trademark of
Dodo Books Indian Ocean Ltd. and OmniScriptum S.R.L publishing group

120 High Road, East Finchley, London, N2 9ED, United Kingdom
Str. Armeneasca 28/1, office 1, Chisinau MD-2012, Republic of Moldova, Europe
Printed at: see last page
ISBN: 978-620-7-78551-3

Contents

Khojamuradov G.M. - Doctor of Medical Sciences, First Deputy Minister of Health and Social Protection of Population of the Republic of Tajikistan

Rasulov S.R. - Doctor of Medical Sciences, Head of the Oncology Department of the State Educational Institution "Institute for Advanced Education in Health Care" of the Republic of Tajikistan

Mirzoev M.Sh. - Doctor of Medical Sciences, Head of the Department of Oral and Maxillofacial Surgery and Paediatric Dentistry of the State Educational Institution "Institute for Advanced Education in Health Care" of the Republic of Tajikistan

Malignant neoplasms of head and neck organs are one of the common cancers in clinical oncology.

The monograph is devoted to the most difficult problem of head and neck tumourigenesis - reconstructive surgical treatment. A critical review of the literature, frequency, prevalence and staging of the tumour process are considered in detail, using our own material. Special attention is paid to the characteristics of defects after surgical interventions, the choice of methods of defect reconstruction depending on the localisation and stage of the disease, immediate and distant results, the parameters of patients' quality of life before and after reconstructive interventions are evaluated.

The book is designed for doctors of oncology, plastic surgeons, maxillofacial surgeons, postgraduates, residents and senior students of medical universities.

Recent decades have been characterised by a steady increase in malignant neoplasms worldwide. Cancer of head and neck organs is one of the common oncological pathologies and accounts for about 3% of the total morbidity structure of malignant neoplasms, and is characterised by a variety of localisations, clinical manifestations, difficulties in the effectiveness of treatment methods and high mortality rates. The predominant morphological variant is squamous cell cancer. A characteristic feature of head and neck cancer is the predominant locoregional spread and high recurrence rate.

The successes achieved in the treatment of early stages of head and neck cancers did not affect the overall 5-year survival rate, which is 65.9%. The choice of treatment tactics is usually based on tumour location, TNM stage of the disease and assessment of possible side effects of treatment. Early stages of squamous cell carcinoma of the head and neck organs are subject to surgical treatment in operable cases or radiation treatment under a radical programme. In cases of locally spreading process, combined and complex approaches are used.

Recent studies have established the advantage of surgical treatment of patients with head and neck cancer at the first stage. However, the key problem in this case is the occurrence of extensive postoperative defects that disturb the basic vital functions, which prompts the search for optimal methods of defect reconstruction, which allows to expand the indications for surgical treatment, providing for one-stage reconstructive and reconstructive operations.

The wide range and combination of treatment methods in the context of complex anatomo-functional features of the head and neck region have specific consequences on the quality of life of patients, including physical, emotional and social dysfunction, which affect the survival rate of patients. This fact gave rise to the tendency to search for and use less massive skin-fascial, mucosa-fascial and skin-muscular grafts, which aims to shorten the operation time, reduce postoperative specific complications and achieve better cosmetic results.

In the book on the basis of own clinical studies, taking into account the latest scientific publications, the frequency, nature and methods of reconstruction of defects after removal of head and neck cancer are highlighted, the frequency of postoperative complications is analysed, the algorithm of choosing the optimal method of plasty depending on the anatomo-topographical characteristics of flaps, localisation and category of complexity of defects is developed, and the immediate and distant results of reconstruction and their influence on the parameters of the quality of life are evaluated.

The monograph is intended for oncologists, plastic and maxillofacial surgeons, postgraduates, clinical residents and will be very useful for senior students of medical universities.

The authors express their sincere gratitude to the staff of the Departments of General Oncology, Radiation and Chemotherapy, Pathomorphology of the Republican Cancer Research Centre (Director - Dr. M.Sc. Huseynzoda Z.H.) for their assistance in performing the clinical study.

__Doctor of Medical Sciences, Professor of the Department of Oncology, Radiation Diagnostics and Radiation Therapy, Abuali Ibni Sino TSMU, Honoured Worker of Tajikistan D.R. Sanginov__

This book is dedicated

To our patients, who by fate are faced with cancer. They entrust their lives in the quest to cure their disease, prolong and improve their quality of life. Every day we learn from them..... Their courage and patience help our perseverance in our work and give us hope for the future. These people hold a special place in our hearts. I am deeply grateful to them for their trust and confidence in our strength and capabilities. Thank you also for permission to use their photographs to illustrate this book.

To all my colleagues and teachers who supported me throughout the whole period of work on it. In particular, to my supervisor - Professor Jumaboy Rakhmatovich Sanginov for his comprehensive support, training and mentoring. Thanks to the life experience of Dzhumaboy Rakhmatovich Sanginov, I have learnt a lot and continue to learn and hope to use his experience in my future life.

And, of course, I dedicate it to my parents and my family members. To them I owe everything. I am grateful for their patience, understanding and support, without which the work on this book would not have been possible.

Candidate of Medical Sciences, head and neck tumour oncologist, assistant of the Department of Oncology, Radiation Diagnostics and Radiation Therapy of Abuali ibni Sino TSMU

I.K. Niyazov

Anatomy of the head and neck is definitely one of the most challenging parts of the science of the human body. Consequently, mastering this clinically relevant and attractive knowledge is one of the most challenging tasks for medical students, subspecialty residents, and practicing physicians. Certainly, the success of any head and neck surgery, among other factors, is directly dependent on the "knowledge factor" of the surgical anatomy of the area.

In the head region are concentrated the main analysers through which a person interacts with the surrounding world. The two main vital - respiratory and digestive systems of the so-called aerodigestive tract originate here. Also, any surgery in the facial area can damage the aesthetics of a person and should be performed taking into account the functional and aesthetic features of this area.

The neck localises major trunk vessels and vital nerves, intraoperative damage to which can be life-threatening. All of the above-mentioned features have caused head and neck surgeons to refer to this area as a "minefield".

The head and neck region has a complex anatomical structure and consists of the following organs and structures:

The pharynx (pharynx) is a wide muscular tube located between the nose, mouth and larynx. The pharynx has three parts - the nasal, oral and laryngeal. From above, the pharynx is attached to the base of the skull (the basilar part of the occipital bone in front of the pharyngeal tubercle). The upper wall of the *pharynx is* called the pharyngeal vault *(fornix pharyngis)*. Below, the pharynx continues into the oesophagus at the level of the 6th-7th cervical vertebra. Posteriorly, the pharynx is bordered by the prevertebral fascia (see neck fascia). The anterior wall is practically absent, because through it the pharynx communicates with the nasal cavity, the oral cavity and the larynx. The pharynx is attached laterally to the medial lamina of the wing spines of the cuneiform bone.

The oropharyngeal space (*spatium peripharyngeum*) is located behind and on the sides of the pharynx. It is divided into: o The pharyngeal space (*spatium retropharyngeum*); lateral pharyngeal space (*sparium lateropharyngeum*).

Nasal pharynx - This is the upper part of the pharynx, located behind the nasal cavity above the lower edge of the palatine curtain.

Oral pharynx - This is the middle part of the pharynx and is connected to the oral cavity through the isthmus of the pharynx. This part of the pharynx is where the airway and digestive tract meet.

Larynx - This is the lower part of the pharynx, located behind the larynx, from the upper edge 18 of the epiglottis to the lower edge of the ring cartilage. The larynx, adjacent to the anterior pharyngeal wall, juts out into the pharyngeal cavity. *Recessus piriformis* (*recessus piriformis*) is formed on the sides of this protrusion.

The pharyngeal wall is formed by the following layers (from inside to outside): *mucosa* (*tunica mucosa*). The mucosa of the nasal part is covered with ciliary epithelium, the lower part - with multilayer neorhoving epithelium. The mucosa contains *pharyngeal* glands (*glandulae pharyngeales*). Submucosal base (*tela submucosa*).

The pharyngeal-basilar fascia (fascia pharyngobasilaris). It is a fibrous lamina, thickest in the upper part.

Muscles of the pharynx. The pharynx has two groups of muscles: longitudinal (dilators) and circular (constrictors). The circular layer of muscles is more developed than the longitudinal one and consists of three *constrictors* - upper, middle and lower (*t. constrictor pharynges superior, medius, inferior*). The upper constrictor begins from the medial lamina of the wing-shaped process of the cuneiform bone and the root of the tongue, the middle - from the horns of the hyoid bone, the lower - from the palpebral and thyroid cartilages of the larynx. Further, the fibres of the constrictors go backwards, and the muscles of the right and left sides meet back to back along the midline, forming the suture of the *pharynx (raphe pharyngis)*.

Longitudinal muscles: The *stylopharyngeus muscle (m.stylopharyngeus)* runs from the styloid process to the pharyngeal wall. It pulls the pharynx upwards and backwards. The palatine pharyngeal muscle and its bundle - the trumpet pharyngeal muscle, which starts from the cartilaginous part of the auditory tube, pulls the pharynx upwards. The pharyngeal fascia covers the outer surface of the pharyngeal constrictors.

The vessels and nerves of the pharynx. In the pharyngeal wall

The ascending pharyngeal artery (from the external carotid artery), pharyngeal branches (from the thyrocervical trunk - branches of the subclavian artery), pharyngeal branches (from the ascending palatine artery - branches of the facial artery) branch off. Venous blood drains through the pharyngeal plexus, then the pharyngeal veins into the internal jugular vein. Lymphatic vessels of the pharynx flow into the pharyngeal and deep lateral (internal jugular) lymph nodes. The pharynx is innervated by branches of the lingual pharyngeal (IX pair) and vagus (X pair) nerves, as well as through the laryngeopharyngeal branches (from the sympathetic trunk), which form a nerve plexus in the pharyngeal wall.

The lymphatic system functions to drain tissue fluid, plasma proteins and other cellular debris back into the bloodstream and is also involved in immune defence. Once this accumulation of substances enters the lymphatic vessels, it is called lymph. The lymph is then filtered by the lymph nodes and sent to the venous system. Knowledge of the anatomy of the lymphatic flow of the head and neck is clinically important.

Lymphatic system of the head and neck

The lymphatic vessels of the head and neck can be divided into two main groups; superficial vessels and deep vessels.

a) Superficial lymphatic vessels - drains lymph from the scalp, face and neck to the superficial ring of lymph nodes at the junction of the neck and head.

б) The deep lymphatic vessels - head and neck arise from the deep cervical lymph nodes. They converge to form the left and right jugular lymphatic trunks:

- Left jugular lymphatic trunk - connects to the thoracic duct at the base of the neck. It enters the venous system via the left subclavian vein.

- Right jugular lymphatic trunk - forms the right lymphatic duct at the base of the neck. It drains into the venous system via the right subclavian vein.

The lymph nodes of the head and neck can be divided into two groups: the superficial ring of lymph nodes and the vertical group of deep lymph nodes.

The superficial lymph nodes receive lymph from the scalp, face and neck. They are arranged in a ring shape; they extend from the chin to the back of the head. They eventually drain into the deep lymph nodes.

Occipital: there are usually 1-3 occipital lymph nodes. They are located at the back of the head at the lateral border of the trapezius muscle and collect lymph from the occipital region of the scalp.

Mastoid: There are usually 2 mastoid lymph nodes, also called posterior lymph nodes. They are located behind the ear and lie at the insertion site of the sternoclavicular-papillary muscle into the mastoid process. They collect lymph from the back of the neck, the upper ear and the back of the external ear canal.

Premaxillary: there are usually 1-3 premaxillary lymph nodes. They are located anterior to the auricle and collect lymph from the superficial areas of the face and temporal region.

Parotid: The parotid lymph nodes are a small group of nodes located superficial to the parotid gland. They collect lymph from the nose, nasal cavity, external ear canal, tympanic cavity and lateral borders of the orbit. Deep in the parotid gland are also the parotid lymph nodes, which drain the nasal cavities and the nasopharynx.

Subchondral: These lymph nodes
are located superficial to the iliac muscle. They collect lymph from the central lower lip, the floor of the mouth and the tip of the tongue.

Submandibular: there are usually between 3-6 submandibular nodes. They are located below the lower jaw in the submandibular triangle and collect lymph from the cheeks, sides of the nose, upper lip, sides of the lower lip, gums and front of the tongue. They also receive lymph from the subcutaneous and facial lymph nodes.

Facial: this group includes the maxillary /suborbital,   cheek and supra-mandibular jaws
lymph nodes. They collect lymph from the mucous membranes of the nose and cheeks, eyelids and conjunctiva.

Superficial cervical: The superficial cervical lymph nodes can be divided into superficial anterior cervical nodes and posterior lateral superficial cervical lymph nodes. The anterior nodes are located close to the anterior jugular vein and collect lymph from the superficial surfaces of the front of the neck.

The posterior lateral nodes are located close to the external jugular vein and collect lymph from the superficial surfaces of the neck (Fig. 1).

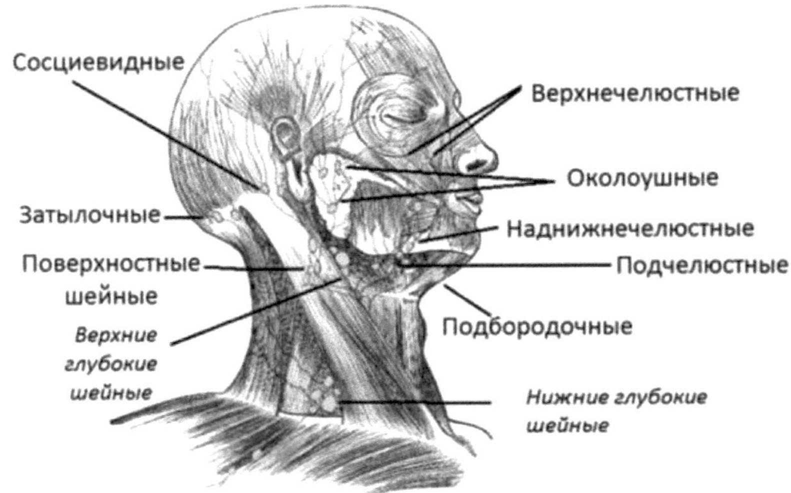

Figure 1. Superficial and deep lymph nodes
of the head and neck.

The deep (cervical) lymph nodes receive all lymph from the head and neck - directly or indirectly via the superficial lymph nodes. They are organised in a vertical chain located in close proximity to the internal jugular vein in the carotid sheath. The outflow vessels from the deep cervical lymph nodes converge to form the jugular lymphatic trunks.

Can be divided into upper and lower deep cervical lymph nodes. There are many of them, but they include the prepharyngeal, pre-tracheal, paratracheal, retropharyngeal, subpharyngeal, jugular-bicepharyngeal (tonsils), jugular- hyoid and supraclavicular nodes (Fig. 2).

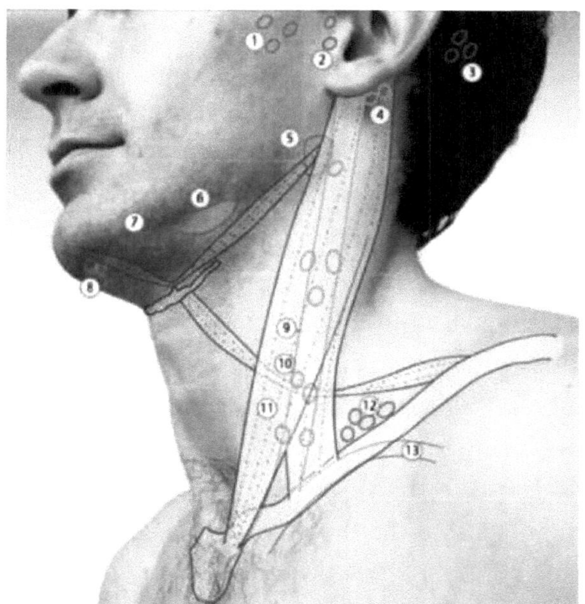

Figure 2. Lymph nodes of the head and neck:
1. parotid, 2. Anterior auricular, 3. Occipital, 4. Papillary, 5. Jugular-biliac (upper deep cervical group), 6. Submandibular salivary gland. 7. Submandibular nodes. 8. Submandibular nodes. 9. Internal jugular nodes. 10. Inferior deep cervical group, 11. Sternoclavicular-papillary, 12.
Supraclavicular nodes. 13. Subclavian vein passing to axillary vein.

Lymph flow from the organs of the head and neck

The lymphatic outflow from the lower lip and mandible goes to the submandibular nodes and to the chin nodes via lymphatic vessels. From the parotid salivary gland lymphatic outflow goes to the parotid lymph nodes. From the hyoid and submandibular salivary glands, lymph drainage occurs to the submandibular lymph nodes. From the teeth of the upper jaw, lymph drainage occurs:

- to the submandibular lymph nodes.
- to the parotid lymph nodes.

- to the occipital lymph nodes.

From the teeth of the lower jaw, lymph flow goes to the submandibular lymph nodes. From the canines and incisors of the upper jaw, lymph flow is to the jawline lymph nodes. From the tongue, lymphatic outflow occurs:

- to the jawline lymph nodes.
- to the submandibular lymph nodes.
- in the pharyngeal lymph nodes.

From all these groups of regional lymph nodes lymph drains to the deep cervical lymph nodes, from which lymph is directed to the right and left jugular trunks.

- **The left jugular trunk** drains lymph from the left side of the head and neck into the thoracic duct.
- **The right** lymphatic **trunk** drains lymph from the right side of the head and neck into the right lymphatic duct. From the right lymphatic and thoracic ducts, lymph then flows to the corresponding right and left venous angles formed by the confluence of the subclavian and internal jugular veins.

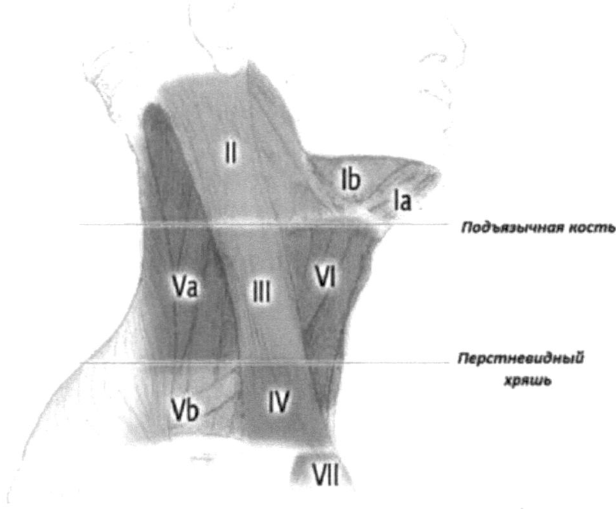

Figure 3. Lymph node levels

Clinical significance of Virchow's node. Virchow's node is a supraclavicular node located in the left supraclavicular fossa (located immediately above the clavicle). It receives lymph drainage from the abdomen. The finding of an enlarged Virchow's node is called Troisier's sign and indicates the presence of cancer in the abdomen, particularly gastric cancer that has spread through the lymphatic vessels.

Pirogov-Waldeyer lymphoid pharyngeal ring

Waldeyer's pharyngeal ring refers to the cluster of lymphatic tissue surrounding the upper part of the pharynx. This lymphatic tissue responds to pathogens that may be ingested or inhaled. It is formed by the tonsils of the pharynx and the isthmus of the pharynx:

1. Right and left palatine tonsils;
2. Right and left tubal tonsils;
3. The pharyngeal tonsil;
4. The lingual tonsil.

The tonsils that make up the ring are as follows:

1. Lingual tonsil - located on the posterior base of the tongue, forming the anterolateral part of the ring.

2. Palatine tonsils - located on each side between the palatine-tongue and palatopharyngeal arches. They are the common 'tonsils' that can be seen in the mouth. They form the side of the ring.

3. Tubal tonsils - these are located where each eustachian tube opens into the nasopharynx and form the side of the ring.

4. The pharyngeal tonsil - also called the nasopharyngeal tonsil /

The adenoid tonsil is located on the roof of the nasopharynx, behind the uvula and forms the posterior-upper part of the ring (Fig. 4).

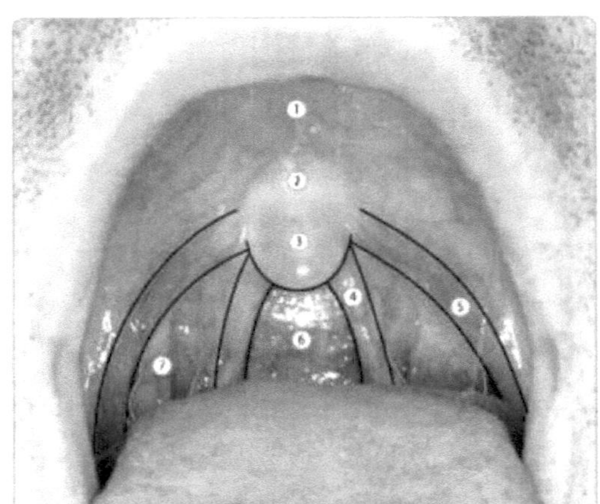

Fig 4. Palatine glands, oropharynx, uvula and palatine
tonsils:

1.Solid Sky. 2. Soft sky. 3. The uvula. 4. The palatopharyngeal arch. 5. Palatine-lingual arch. 6. Posterior wall of the oropharynx. 7. Boundaries of the location of the palatine tonsils (green line).

Clinical significance: inflammation of the tonsils (tonsillitis)

The palatine tonsils may become inflamed due to a viral or bacterial infection. In this case, they appear red and enlarged and are accompanied by enlargement of the jugular lymph nodes. Chronic infection of the palatine tonsils can be treated by removing them, tonsillectomy. When performing tonsillectomy, there may be bleeding primarily from the external palatine vein and secondarily from the tonsil branch of the facial artery.

If the infection spreads to the peritonsillar tissue, it can cause an abscess to form. It can

cause a deviation of the uvula known as sore throat, which can be complicated by swelling and closure of the pharynx. This complication is treated with drainage of the abscess and antibiotics (Figure 5).

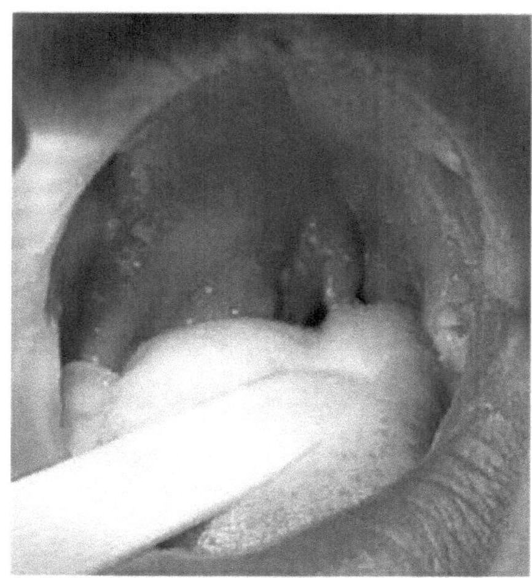

Figure 5. Angina - inflammation of peritonsillar tissue, uvula deviated to the right as a result of inflammation.

Lymph drainage of the brain

Lymphatic vessels in the brain were thought to be absent until scientists discovered lymphatic vessels in the brains of mice and then humans in 2015. Work is underway to identify and characterise the lymphatic vessels involved.

Anomalies of the pharynx

Soft palate incompleteness - which leads to impaired swallowing (ingestion of food and liquid into the nasopharynx and nasal cavity) and speech function (open nasality). Examination reveals a sagittal cleft of the soft palate in the middle of it, often the uvula is absent or, conversely, bifurcated. The treatment of this anomaly is surgical - soft palate plasty.

Failure **to close the second gill slit** and formation of a branching canal leading from the supramandibular fossa into the soft palate. This canal is of some importance in the pathogenesis of paratonsillar abscesses.

Middle and lateral fistulas (cysts) of the neck. These passages originate in the pharynx and extend into the lower neck.

The middle canal is from the root of the tongue through the body of the hyoid bone to the thyroid gland. It forms the median cyst of the neck if it is not closed.

The lateral canal originates in the pear-shaped sinus of the larynopharynx and runs down along the sternoclavicular-axillary muscle, from which a lateral neck cyst can form. Both cysts may manifest themselves after an infection or trauma to the neck, when a tumour-like mass appears, painless, mobile, gradually increasing in size. It usually festered and emptied through a fistula in the skin.

Arteries of the head and neck

The common carotid artery *(a. carotis communis)* branches from the brachial trunk on the right and from the aortic arch on the left. The length of the right artery is 6-12 cm, the left artery is 2-3 cm longer. The common carotid artery lies behind the sternoclavicular-axillary and scapulohyoid muscles and follows vertically upwards in front of the transverse processes of the cervical vertebrae without giving off any branches along the way.

The common carotid artery can be palpated and, if necessary, pressed against the carotid tubercle on the transverse process of the VI cervical vertebra lateral to the lower larynx.

The right common carotid artery (*a. carotis communis dextra*) branches from the brachiocephalic trunk, while the left common carotid artery branches from the aortic arch. In this connection, the left common carotid artery is 2.5-3 cm longer than the right one. At the level of the sternoclavicular articulations, the common carotid arteries exit to the neck. In the neck, the arteries are located in the large interfascial gap, which is delimited medially by the trachea and oesophagus, posteriorly by the anterior vertebral fascia and anterior ladder muscle, and laterally and anteriorly by the sternoclavicular-papillary muscle. In the neck, the common carotid arteries are part of the neurovascular bundle, which includes, in addition to the common carotid artery, the internal jugular vein, and the vagus nerve. As a rule, the common carotid artery does not give branches, but in some cases (especially with a high variant of bifurcation), the superior thyroid artery may branch from its upper part 0.2-1.5 cm below the bifurcation.

The external carotid artery rises in the neck to the temporomandibular joint, where it divides into its terminal branches: the maxillary and superficial temporal arteries. All its branches supply blood to the organs and partially to the muscles of the neck, soft tissues of the face and the whole head, walls of the nasal cavity, walls and organs of the oral cavity. The branches of the external carotid artery run as if along the radii of the circle corresponding to the head and can be divided into three groups of three arteries each: anterior, middle and posterior groups (Fig. b).

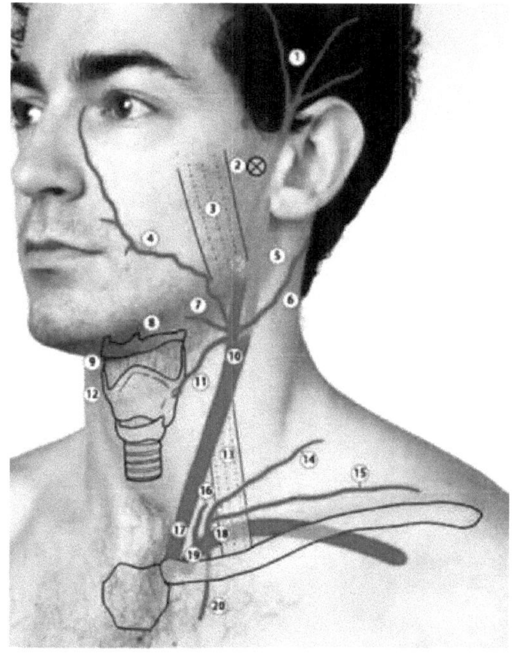

Figure 6. Arteries of the face and neck:
1. Superficial temporal artery. 2. The maxillary artery. 3. Chewing artery. 4. Facial artery. 5. Internal carotid artery. 6. Occipital artery. 7. Lingual artery. 8. The greater horn of the hyoid bone. 9. Hyoid hyoid membrane.   10. Bifurcation of the carotid artery. 11. Upper hyoid.
thyroid artery. 12. Adam's apple. 13. Anterior ladder muscle. 14. Transverse cervical artery. 15. Supra scapular artery. 16. Vertebral artery. 17. Common carotid artery. 18. Scutellar trunk. 19. Subclavian artery. 20. Internal thoracic artery.

The front group includes:
- the superior thyroid artery, which supplies blood to the thyroid gland, larynx;
- lingual artery - tongue, palatine tonsils, mucous membrane of the oral cavity;
- facial artery - soft tissues of the face, mimic muscles.

The rear group includes:
- occipital artery, which supplies blood to the muscles of the back of the head, the auricle, and the dura mater;
- posterior auricular - the skin of the back of the head, the auricle and the tympanic cavity;
- the sternoclavicular-axillary artery to the muscle of the same name.

The middle group includes:
- the ascending pharyngeal artery;
- the maxillary artery;
- superficial temporal artery. All of them supply blood to their respective areas of the head and neck.

The facial artery (*a. facialis*) branches from the external carotid artery at the level of the angle of the mandible, 3-5 mm above the lingual artery. In the area of the submandibular triangle, the facial artery adjoins the submandibular gland (or passes through it), then bends over the edge of the mandible to the face (in front of the masseter muscle) and goes upwards and forwards, towards the corner of the mouth, and then to the area of the medial corner of the eye.

The following branches branch from the facial artery:

1) *The ascending palatine artery (a. palatina ascendens)* from the initial part of the facial artery, runs up the lateral wall of the pharynx, penetrates between the pharyngeal and pharyngeal muscles and supplies them with blood). The final branches of the artery are directed to the palatine tonsil, the pharyngeal part of the auditory tube, and the pharyngeal mucosa;

2) *The tonsillar branch (r. tonsillaris)* goes up the lateral pharyngeal wall to the palatine tonsil, pharyngeal wall, root of the tongue;

3) *The submental artery (a. submentalis)* follows the outer surface of the maxillary hyoid muscle to the chin and neck muscles above the hyoid bone.

On the face, in the area of the corner of the mouth, come off:

4) *lower lip artery (a. labialis inferior)* and 5) *upper lip artery (a. labialis superior)*. Both arteries run into the lip thickness and anastomose with similar arteries of the opposite side;

6) the *angular artery (a. angularis)* is the terminal branch of the facial artery and runs to the medial corner of the eye. Here it anastomoses with the dorsal nasal artery, a branch of the ocular artery (from the internal carotid artery system).

The maxillary **artery** (*a. maxillaris)* is also the terminal branch of the external carotid artery. The initial part of the artery is covered on the lateral side by the mandibular branch. The artery reaches (at the level of the lateral wing muscle) to the subscapularis and then to the fossa palatina, where it splits into its terminal branches. According to the topography of the maxillary artery, three sections are distinguished in it:

maxillary, wing and wing palatine. The following arteries branch from the maxillary artery within its maxillary section:

1) *The deep auricular artery (a. auricularis profunda)* goes to the temporomandibular joint, the external ear canal and the tympanic membrane;

2) *The anterior tympanic artery (a. tympanica anterior)* follows through the stony ty*mpanic* cleft of the temporal bone to the mucous membrane of the tympanic cavity;

3) *The inferior alveolar artery (a. alveolaris inferior)* is a large artery that enters the mandibular canal and gives off dental branches on its way. This artery leaves the canal through the jawline as the chin artery, which branches in the mimic muscles and in the skin of the chin

4) *The middle meningeal artery (a. meningea media) is the* largest of all arteries feeding the dura mater. This artery penetrates into the cranial cavity through the spinous opening of the large wing of the cuneiform bone, gives off the upper tympanic artery, which goes through the canal of the muscle that stretches the tympanic membrane to the mucous membrane of the tympanic cavity, as well as frontal and parietal branches to the dura mater.

Within the **wing section,** branches feeding the masseter muscles branch off the maxillary artery:

1) *the masseter artery* goes to the muscle of the same name;

2) *the anterior and posterior deep temporal arteries* go into the thickness of the temporalis muscle;

3) *The wing branches* go to the muscles of the same name;

4) *The cheek artery is* directed to the cheek muscle and the cheek mucosa;

5) *The posterior superior alveolar artery* penetrates the maxillary sinus through the same-named holes in the maxillary tubercle and supplies blood to its mucous membrane, while its

dental branches supply blood to the teeth and gums of the maxilla.

From the third, the **wing palate.**

The maxillary artery has three terminal branches:

1) the suborbital artery (a. infraorbitalis) passes into the eye socket through the lower eye slit, where it branches to the lower rectus and oblique muscles of the eye. Then, through the suborbital opening, this artery exits through the canal of the same name to the face and supplies blood to the mimic muscles located in the thickness of the upper lip, in the area of the nose and lower eyelid, and the skin covering them. Here the suborbital artery anastomoses with branches of the facial and superficial temporal arteries

2) the descending palatine artery (a. palatina descendens) supplies blood to the hard and soft palate via the greater and lesser palatine arteries, gives off the cuneiform palatine artery, which passes through the orifice of the same name into the nasal cavity, and the lateral posterior nasal arteries and posterior septal branches to the nasal mucosa.

Anterior superior alveolar arteries, *aa. alveolares superiores anteriores,* which run through the canals in the external wall of the maxillary sinus and supply blood to the teeth of the maxilla, the gingiva and the mucous membrane of the maxillary sinus. The inferior alveolar artery (mandibular branch of the terminal branch group) is directed downwards between the mandibular branch and the medial wing muscle into the mandibular canal. It supplies blood to the mandible, teeth and gums. Its terminal branch exits through the orifice of the same name to the chin, where it anastamoses with branches of the facial artery. The teeth, periodontium, gingiva, alveolar process of the jaws are supplied with blood through the maxillary artery, which gives off branches: the inferior alveolar artery, the posterior superior alveolar artery and the suborbital artery, from which the anterior superior alveolar arteries and dental branches branch off. The posterior *superior alveolar artery* (*a. alveolaris superior posterior*) originates at the transition of the maxillary artery into the maxillary fossa behind the maxillary tubercle. Through the posterior superior alveolar foramen it penetrates into the bone; it divides into dental branches, passing together with the posterior superior alveolar nerves into the alveolar canals in the posterolateral wall of the maxilla to the roots of the upper large molars. *Peri-dental branches* branch from the dental *branches* to the tissues surrounding the roots of the teeth. The periodontium is a complex of tissues that includes the root cementum, periodontal ligament and alveolar bone. The periodontal ligament has a rich blood supply. The main sources of blood supply are the alveolar arteries. Individual branches reach the apical periodontium and ascend in a crown direction before penetrating the dental pulp, while gingival arterioles penetrate the periodontal ligament, spreading in an apical direction. In addition, a large number of vessels penetrate the periodontal ligament through bony foramen. Thus, unlike the dental pulp, the periodontium has a rich collateral circulation. The capillary network is also well developed. It is more pronounced in the area of bone tissue than at the root surface. In the vicinity of the vessels there are lymphatic capillaries that carry lymph to the regional lymph nodes.

Venous system of the head and neck

Sinuses of the dura mater. The sinuses (sinuses) of the dura mater, formed by splitting the dura mater into two laminae, are channels through which venous blood flows from the brain to the internal jugular veins. Sheets of the dura mater, forming the sinus, are tightly stretched and do not collapse. Therefore, on the cut sinuses gaping; sinuses do not have valves. This structure of the sinuses allows venous blood to flow freely from the brain regardless of fluctuations in intracranial pressure. On the inner surfaces of the bones of the skull, at the location of the sinuses of the dura mater, there are corresponding furrows. The following dura mater sinuses are distinguished (Fig. 7).

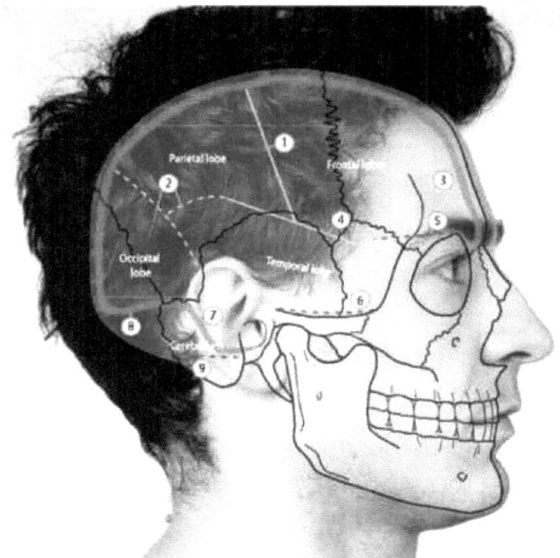

Figure 7. Venous sinuses and cerebral lobes:
1. The central furrow. 2. Suggested division between the lobes of the brain (green line). 3. Upper sagittal sinus. 4. Lateral sulcus of the brain. 5. Anterior cranial fossa (red line). 6. Level of the middle cranial fossa (red line). 7. Sigmoid sinus. 8 Transverse sinus. 9. Level of the posterior cranial fossa.

1. *The superior sagittal sinus (sinus sagittalis superior) is* located along the entire outer (upper) edge of the sickle of the large brain, from the cockscomb of the lattice bone to the internal occipital protrusion. In its anterior parts, this sinus has anastomoses with the veins of the nasal cavity. The posterior end of the sinus flows into the transverse sinus. To the right and left of the superior sagittal sinus there are lateral lacunae

communicating with it. These are small cavities between the outer and inner layers (sheets) of the dura mater, the number and size of which are very variable. The lacunar cavities communicate with the upper sagittal sinus cavity, and the dura mater veins, cerebral veins and diploid veins flow into them.

2. *The inferior sagittal sinus (sinus sagittalis inferior)* is located in the thickness of the lower free edge of the cerebral *sulcus*; it is much smaller than the superior sinus. With its posterior end, the inferior sagittal sinus flows into the straight sinus, in its anterior part, at the place where the lower edge of the cerebral sulcus meets the anterior edge of the cerebellar plaque.

3. *Straight sinus (sinus rectus),* located sagittally in the cleft of the cerebellar peduncle along the line of attachment of the cerebellar sickle. The rectus sinus connects the posterior ends of the superior and inferior sagittal sinuses. In addition to the inferior sagittal sinus, the great cerebral vein flows into the anterior end of the straight sinus. Posteriorly, the straight sinus flows into the transverse sinus, into its middle part, called the sinus drain. The posterior part of the superior sagittal sinus and the occipital sinus also enter here.

4. *The transverse sinus (sinus transversus),* lies in the place where the cerebellar capitulum departs from the dura mater. On the inner surface of the scales of the occipital bone, a broad furrow of the transverse sinus corresponds to this sinus. The place where the superior sagittal, occipital and straight sinuses flow into it is called the sinus drain (confluence of the sinuses). On the right and left side, the transverse sinus continues into the sigmoid sinus of the respective side,

5. *The occipital sinus (sinus occipitalis)* lies at the base of the cerebellar sulcus. Descending along the internal occipital ridge, it reaches the posterior edge of the greater occipital foramen,

where it divides into two branches covering the back and sides of the foramen. Each branch of the occipital sinus flows into the sigmoid sinus of its side, and its upper end into the transverse sinus.

6. *The sigmoid sinus (sinus sigmoideus)* (paired), located in the *sulcus of the* same name on the inner surface of the skull, is S-shaped. In the area of the jugular foramen, the sigmoid sinus passes into the internal jugular vein.

7. *The cavernous sinus (sinus cavernosus),* paired, is located at the base of the skull, lateral to the Turkish saddle. The internal carotid artery and some cranial nerves pass through this sinus. This sinus has a very complex construction in the form of communicating with each other caves, in connection with which it received its name. Between the right and left cavernous sinuses there are communications (anastomoses) in the form of anterior and posterior inter cavernous sinuses, which are located in the thickness of the diaphragm of the Turkish saddle, in front of and behind the pituitary gland. The anterior cavernous sinus is joined by the parietal cuneiform sinus and the superior ocular vein.

8. *Cuneiform-parietal sinus (sinus sphenoparietalis),* paired, adjoins the free posterior margin of the small wing of the cuneiform bone, in the cleft of the dura attached here.

9. *The upper and lower stony sinuses (sinus petrosus superior et sinus petrosus inferior),* paired, lie along the upper and lower edges of the temporal bone pyramid. Both sinuses take part in the formation of venous blood outflow pathways from the cavernous sinus to the sigmoid sinus. The right and left inferior stony sinuses are connected by several veins lying in the cleavage of the dura in the area of the occipital bone body, which are called the basilar plexus. This plexus connects to the internal vertebral venous plexus through the greater occipital

foramen.

Diploid veins. In the cancellous substance of the bones of the cranial *vault*, the *diploicae*, bone canals are formed that become *vv.* diploicae; most diploic veins extend from the top down to the base of the skull, where they may connect through openings in the cranial bones either to the subcutaneous veins of the cranial vault or to the venous sinuses of the dura mater. There are connections of superficial veins of the vault directly with venous sinuses. The following diploic veins are distinguished:

1) *frontal (v. diploica frontalis)*;

2) anterior and posterior temporal (*vv. diploicae temporales anterior et posterior*);

3) occipital (*v. diploica occipitalis*). They are located in the bones corresponding to their names.

Emissary veins. The veins of the scalp are connected to the veins of the skull by the emissary veins.

The parietal emissary vein (*v. emissaria parietalis*) connects the superficial temporal vein to the posterior temporal diploid vein and to the superior sagittal sinus via the parietal foramen.

The mastoid emissary vein (*v. emissaria mastoidea*) passes through the mastoid foramen and connects the occipital vein and the posterior temporal diploid vein to the sigmoid sinus.

The condylar emissary vein (*v. emissaria condilaris*) penetrates the cond*ylar* canal and forms an anastomosis between the vertebral venous plexuses and the deep vein of the neck.

The occipital emissary vein (*v. emissaria occipitalis*) is located in the opening of the external occipital protrusion; it connects the occipital vein to the occipital diploid vein and the transverse sinus.

Superficial and deep veins of the head and neck

The internal *jugular* **vein** (*v. Jugularis interna*) is a large vessel that, like the external jugular vein, collects blood from the head and neck, from the areas corresponding to the branching of the external and internal carotid and vertebral arteries.

The internal jugular vein is a direct continuation of the sigmoid sinus of the dura mater. It begins at the level of the jugular foramen, below which there is a small dilation - the upper bulb of the internal jugular vein. At first, the vein runs behind the internal carotid artery, then laterally. Even lower, the vein is located behind the common carotid artery in a common with it and the vagus nerve connective tissue (fascial) sheath. Above the place of confluence with the subclavian vein, the internal jugular vein has a second extension - the lower bulb of the internal jugular vein, and above and below the bulb - one valve each. Through the sigmoid sinus, from which the internal jugular vein originates, venous blood flows from the system of sinuses of the dura mater. The superficial and deep brain veins - diploid veins, as well as the ocular veins and labyrinth veins - flow into these sinuses and can be considered as intracranial tributaries of the internal jugular vein (Fig. 8).

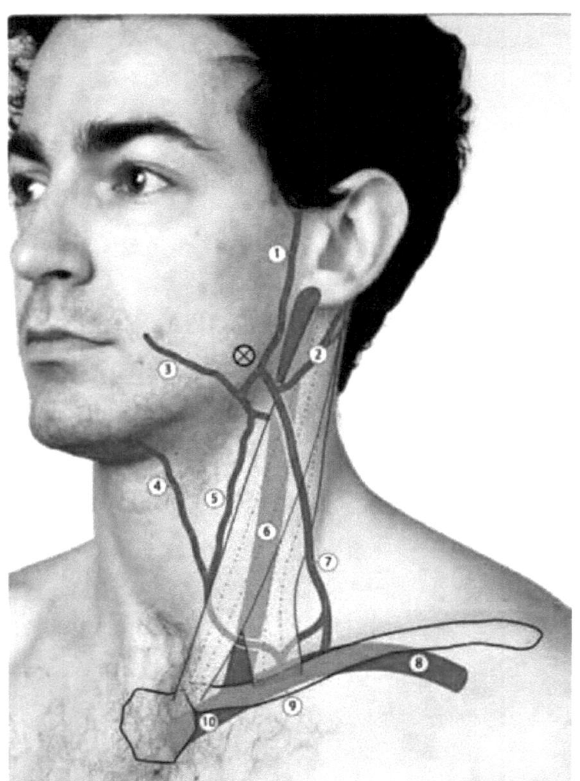

Figure 8. Superficial and deep veins of the face and neck. 1. Retromandibular vein. 2. Posterior auricular vein. 3. Facial vein. 4. Anterior jugular vein. 5. Communicating vein. 6. Internal jugular vein. 7. External jugular vein. 8. Axillary vein. 9. Subclavian vein. 10. Left brachiofemoral vein.

The diploic veins (vv. diploicae) are valveless, through which blood flows away from the bones of the skull. In the cranial cavity, these veins communicate with meningeal veins and sinuses of the dura mater, and externally with the veins of the external coverings of the head by means of emissary veins. The largest diploid veins are the frontal diploid vein, which flows into the superior sagittal sinus, the anterior temporal diploid vein into the cuneiform parietal sinus, the posterior temporal diploid vein into the mastoid emissary vein, and the occipital diploid vein into the transverse sinus or occipital emissary vein.

The sinuses of the dura mater connect to the veins located in the outer covering of the head by means of the emissary veins.

The emissary veins are located in small bony canals, through which blood flows from the sinuses to the outside, i.e. to the veins that collect blood from the exterior of the head. The *parietal emissary vein,* which passes through the parietal foramen of the eponymous bone and connects the superior sagittal sinus with the external veins of the head, is distinguished. The mastoid emissary *vein is* located in the canal of the mastoid process of the temporal bone. The condyle *emissary vein* enters through the condyle canal of the occipital bone. The parietal and mastoid emissary veins connect the sigmoid sinus with the tributaries of the occipital vein, and the condyle emissary vein also connects with the veins of the external vertebral plexus.

The upper and lower *ophthalmic* **veins** (*vv. ophthdlmicae superior et inferior*) are valveless. The first of them, the larger one, contains the veins of the nose and forehead, upper eyelid, lattice bone, lacrimal gland, membranes of the eyeball and most of its muscles. The upper ocular vein in the area of the medial corner of the eye anastomoses with the **facial vein** (*v. facialis*). The inferior ocular vein is formed from the veins of the lower eyelid, neighbouring muscles of the eye, lies on the lower wall of the eye socket under the optic nerve and flows into the superior ocular vein, which exits the eye socket through the superior ocular slit and flows into the cavernous sinus.

The veins of the *labyrinth* (*vv. labyrinthi*) exit the *labyrinth* through the internal auditory canal and flow into the nearby inferior stony sinus.

Extracranial tributaries of the internal jugular vein:

1) pharyngeal veins (vv. pharyngedles) are unvalved and carry blood from the pharyngeal **plexus,** which is located on the posterior surface of the pharynx. Venous blood from the pharynx, auditory tube, soft palate and occipital part of the dura mater drains into this plexus;

2) The lingual vein (v. lingualis), which is formed by the dorsal veins of the tongue (*vv. dorsales linguae)*, the deep vein of the tongue (v. *profunda linguae)* and the hyoid vein (*v. sublingualis)*;

3) the superior thyroid vein (v. thyroidea superior) sometimes flows into the facial vein, is adjacent to the artery of the same name, and has valves. The superior *laryngeal vein (v. laryngea superior)* and the *sternocleidomastoid vein (v. sternocleidomastoidea*) flow into the superior thyroid vein. In some cases, one of the thyroid veins zidetes laterally to the internal jugular vein and flows into it independently as the *middle thyroid vein (v. thyroidea media)*;

4) The facial vein (v. facialis) flows into the internal jugular vein at the level of the hyoid bone. Smaller veins formed in the soft tissues of the face flow into it: angular vein (*v. angularis*), supraorbital vein, veins of the upper and lower eyelids, external nasal veins, upper and lower lip veins, external palatine vein, chin vein, parotid veins, deep facial vein;

5) The mandibular vein (v. retromandibularis) is a large vessel. It runs in front of the auricle, passes through the parotid gland behind the mandibular branch (to the outside of the external carotid artery), and flows into the internal jugular vein. The anterior ear veins, superficial, middle and deep temporal veins, veins of the temporomandibular joint, wing plexus, into which the middle meningeal veins, parotid gland veins and middle ear veins flow, bring blood to the mandibular vein.

The external *jugular* **vein** (*v. jugularis externa*) is formed at the anterior edge of the sternoclavicular-papillary muscle by the confluence of its two tributaries - the anterior one, which is an anastomosis with the mandibular vein flowing into the internal jugular vein, and the posterior one formed by the confluence of the occipital and posterior auricular veins. The external jugular vein runs down the anterior surface of the sternoclavicular-papillary muscle to the clavicle, penetrates the anterotracheal plate of the cervical fascia and flows into the angle of confluence of the subclavian and internal jugular veins or common trunk with the latter into the subclavian vein. At the level of its mouth and in the middle of the neck, this vein has two paired valves. The *supra scapular vein* and *transverse neck veins* flow into the external jugular vein.

The anterior jugular **vein** (*v. jugularis* anterior) is formed from the small veins of the chin, runs downwards in the anterior region of the neck, penetrates the anterotracheal plate of the cervical fascia, and penetrates the interfascial supraglottic space. In this space, the left and right anterior jugular veins are connected by a transverse anastomosis forming the **jugular venous arch.** This arc flows into the external jugular vein on the right and left sides.

The subclavian **vein** (*v. subclavia) is* an unpaired trunk, is a continuation of the axillary vein, runs ahead of the anterior ladder muscle from the lateral edge of the I rib to the sternoclavicular joint, behind which it connects with the internal jugular vein. At the beginning and at the end of the subclavian vein has valves, the vein has no permanent tributaries. The thoracic veins and the dorsal scapular vein flow into the subclavian vein most often.

Cranial nerves

*I pair. **Olfactory nerve, n. olphactorius** -* no nuclei, is an outgrowth of the brain. By function - specific sensitivity, olfaction. Exit from the brain - olfactory bulbs (hypothalamus, intermediate brain). Exit from the skull - pierced plate of the lattice bone. The nerve represents 15-20 olfactory filaments. The zone of innervation is the mucous membrane of the upper nasal passage and the upper nasal shell (olfactory area).

II pair. Optic nerve, n. opticus - No nuclei, is an outgrowth of the brain. By function - specific sensitivity, vision. Exits the brain through the optic junction (hypothalamus, intermediate brain). Exits the skull through the optic canal. The nerve has four parts: ocular, ocular, tubule and cranial and has the same sheaths as the brain. The area of innervation is the retina (rods and cones).

III pair. Oculomotor nerve, n. oculomotorius - nuclei - motor nucleus of the oculomotor nerve, dorsal central nucleus of Perlia, supplementary nucleus of Jakubowicz. Exits the brain through the interfossa fossa. In the cranial cavity passes through the cavernous sinus. Exits the skull through the upper ocular fissure. Zone of innervation: Motor fibres innervate: muscles of the eyeball: the muscle raising the upper eyelid, the upper rectus muscle, medial and lower rectus and inferior oblique muscles. Autonomic fibres: The bodies of the first neurons lie in the nuclei
Perlia and Jakubovich. The axons of the first neurons as part of the nerve go into the eye socket, separate and go to the ciliary ganglion, where they switch to the bodies of the second neurons. Axons of two neurons go further as part of the short ciliary nerves of the 5th pair and innervate the ciliary muscle of the eye and the sphincter of the pupil. Signs of III pair lesion:
- eyelid ptosis (blepharoptosis),
- dilated pupil (mydriasis),
- Diplopia (double vision),
- divergent strabismus (strobismus).

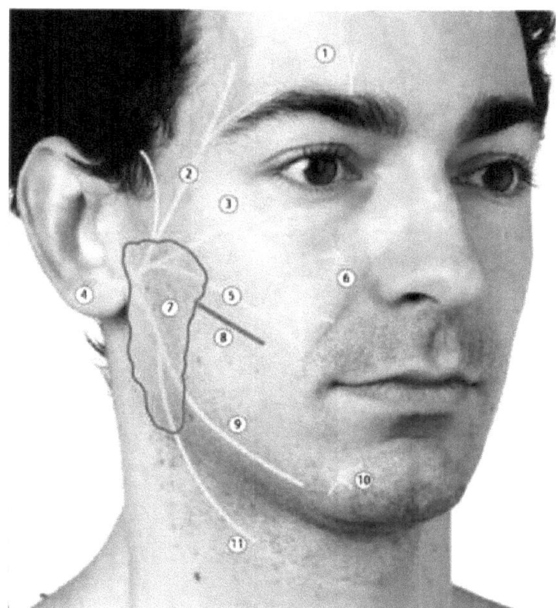

Figure 9. Facial and trigeminal nerves, parotid salivary gland. 1. Supraorbital nerve. 2. Facial nerve: temporal branch. 3. Facial nerve: zygomatic branch. 4. Stem of the facial nerve. 5. Facial nerve: cheek branches. 6. Suborbital nerve. 7. Parotid salivary gland (green lines). 8. The duct of the parotid gland. 9. Facial nerve: marginal mandibular branch. 10. Chin nerve. 11. Cervical branches of the facial nerve.

Muscle structure of the face and neck

The neck muscles are a large array of superficial, medial and deep muscles. The neck muscles are mainly responsible for bending and other movements of the head in all directions. In addition, they perform several other functions: keeping the head in balance, helping with swallowing and pronouncing sounds. The neck muscles are closely connected to a number of important structures and, unlike the facial muscles, are covered by dense fascia.

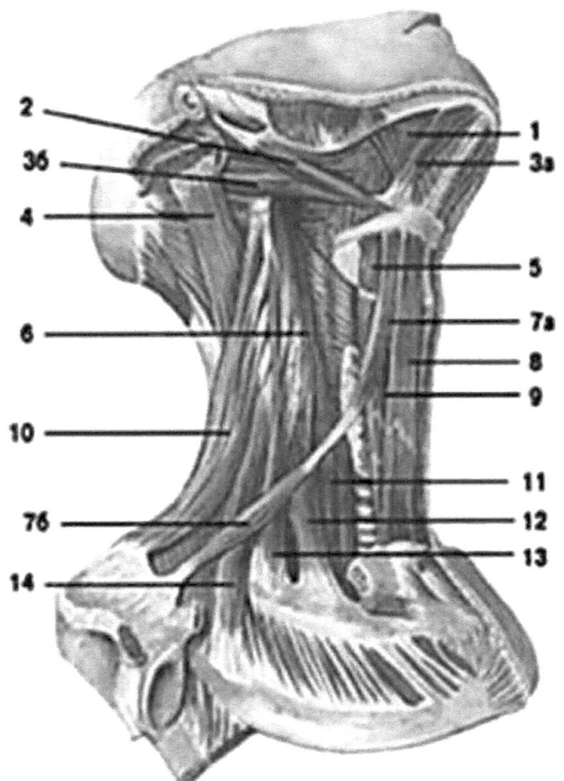

Figure 10: Muscles of the neck. 1. Jaw hyoid muscle. 2. The hyoid hyoid muscle. 3. Biceps muscle: a) anterior abdominis. b) posterior abdominis. 4. The longest muscle of the head. 5. The thyroid hyoid muscle. 6. Long muscle of the head. 7. Scapulohyoid muscle: a) upper abdomen, b) lower abdomen. 8. Sternal hyoid muscle. 9. Muscle that lifts the scapula. 11. Long muscle of the neck. 12. Anterior ladder muscle. 13. Middle ladder muscle. 14. Posterior ladder muscle.

Superficial muscles of the neck. The superficial muscle group consists of two parts: the saphenous muscle and the sternoclavicular-papillary muscle.

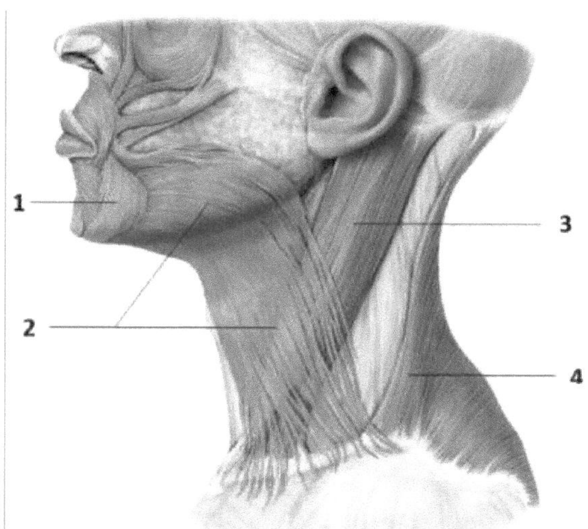

Figure 11. Superficial muscles of the neck: 1. Muscle lowering the corner of the mouth. 2. Platysma. 3. Sternoclavicular-papillary. 4. Trapezius muscle (cervical part).

The sternoclavicular muscle is a long belt muscle with two heads. The muscle comes from the sternal head (the anterior surface of the sternum) and the clavicular head (the upper surface of the middle third of the clavicle). Its attachment site is the mastoid process of the temporal bone, or rather the outer surface of this process.

If both halves contract, the muscle pulls the head forward and bends the neck. When you take a deep breath, it lifts your ribs and sternum upwards. If one half is contracted, the muscle tilts the head forward on the side of the contraction. It is responsible for turning the head upwards and to the opposite side.

The saphenous muscle is located (*m. platysma colli*) just under the skin and is flat and thin. It starts in the chest below the clavicle, runs medially and upwards, covering almost the entire anterolateral neck. Only a small triangle-shaped area above the jugular notch remains uncovered.

Bundles of the saphenous muscle rise into the facial region, woven into the masseteric fascia. Some of them join the laughing muscle and the muscle that lowers the lower lip. This muscle pulls back the skin and protects the veins from being squeezed. It can also pull the corners of the mouth down, which is important for a person's facial expressions.

The middle or medial muscles of the neck. This group of muscles includes: lateral and medial wing muscles, cheek muscle, midline, anterior and posterior ladder muscles, biceps, thyroid, sternocleidomastoid, sternothyroid and trapezius muscles.

The maxillary hyoid muscle has the shape of an irregular triangle and is flat. It starts in the region of the lower jaw, where the maxillary hyoid line is located. The bundles of the muscle run from top to bottom and from back to front. When they reach the midline, they join the bundles of the same muscle on the opposite side to form the suture of the maxillary hyoid muscle. The posterior fascicles attach to the anterior portion of the hyoid bone. The left and right maxillary hyoid muscles form the floor of the mouth and are called the diaphragm of the mouth.

The main task of the jaw hyoid muscle is to lift the hyoid bone upwards. If the muscle is fixed, it helps to lower the mobile (lower) jaw and is an antagonist to the masseter muscles. If the muscle is contracted during eating, it lifts and presses the tongue against the palate, allowing food to pass into the pharynx (Figure 12).

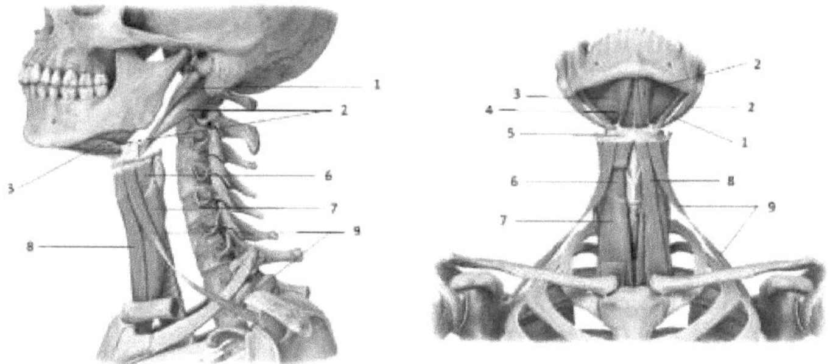

Fig. 12: Group of supra- and subgluteal muscles of the neck: 1. Sciatic hyoid. 2. The bicuspid. 3. Jaw hyoid. 4. Sublingual suture. 5. The hyoid bone. 6. Thyroid- hyoid.   7. Hyoid-sublingual.   8. Sternothoracic.
hyoid. 9. Scapulo-sublingual.

The biceps muscle is the tendon that connects the posterior and anterior abdomen, attached to the greater horn and the body of the hyoid bone by a fascial loop. The biceps muscle helps with active opening of the mouth (with resistance, for example) by lowering the lower jaw when the hyoid bone is fixed. When swallowing, it lifts the hyoid bone towards the mastoid process and the mandible (if the latter is fixed by the masseter muscles). The hyoid hyoid muscle has a thin, flattened abdomen starting at the temporal bone styloid process, running forwards and downwards, located along the biceps muscle (anterior surface of its posterior abdomen). The distal end of the muscle splits, covers the tendon of the biceps muscle with legs, attaches to the greater horn, the body of the hyoid bone and plays an important role in the process of articulate speech.

The sternocleidomastoid muscle is located deep. The function of the muscle is to lower the hyoid bone. When the supra hyoid muscles (located between the mobile jaw and hyoid bone) contract, the sterno hyoid muscle, together with the mandibular, sternocleidomastoid muscle, moves the lower jaw.

The hyoid-sublingual muscle starts near the jawline of the mandible, then runs downwards and backwards. It is located higher up from the maxillary hyoid muscle and attaches to the body of the hyoid bone (its anterior surface).

Lifts the hyoid bone upwards. When fixed, it helps to lower the mobile jaw, making it an antagonist of the masseter muscles.

The scapulohyoid muscle is a member of the sub hyoid muscle group and is a paired muscle of the anterior surface of the neck. It has a long flattened shape and a tendon that divides it into two abdomens. It pulls the hyoid bone downwards and provides tension to the pretracheal plate of the cervical fascia.

The sternocleidomastoid muscle has a flat shape. It originates from the posterior surface of the first cartilage and the handle of the sternum, goes upwards and attaches to the thyroid cartilage of the larynx (the oblique line of its lateral surface). The main task of this muscle is to lower the larynx.

The hyoid muscle starts from the oblique line of the thyroid cartilage. It is attached to the greater horn, body of the hyoid bone. Lifts the larynx when the hyoid bone is fixed.

The deep muscles of the neck are a complex of lateral and medial (prevertebral) muscles. The list of deep tissues includes the anterior, posterior, middle ladder muscles, long neck muscle, lateral rectus, anterior rectus and long head muscles (Fig. 13).

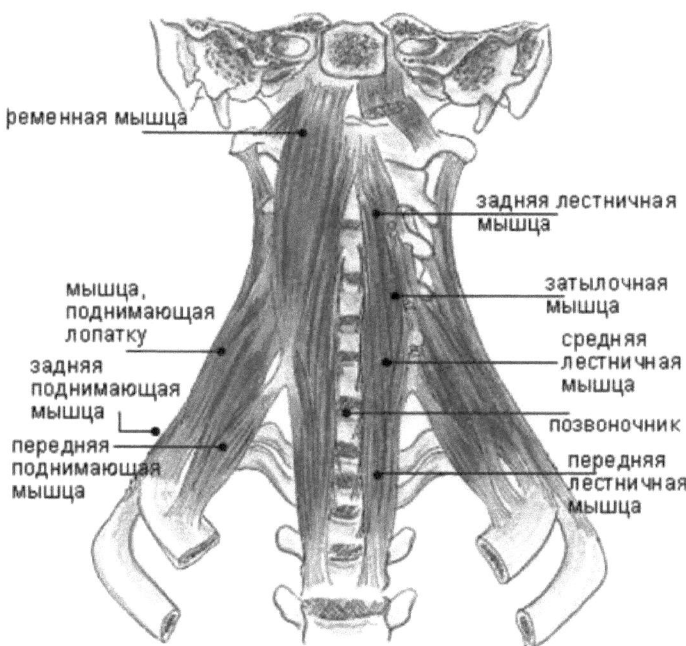

Figure 13: The deep muscle group of the neck.

The anterior ladder muscle originates from the anterior tubercles of the third and fourth cervical vertebrae, runs downwards and forwards, attaches to the anterior ladder muscle of the first rib in front of the subclavian artery sulcus.

This muscle occupies an important place in the functioning of the body. It provides lifting of the upper rib during breathing, rotation of the neck in different directions, forward bending of the cervical part of the spinal column.

The middle ladder muscle starts at the posterior tubercles of the six lower vertebrae of the neck, runs down behind the anterior ladder muscle and attaches to the upper surface of the 1st rib, behind the subclavian artery sulcus. The middle ladder muscle acts as an inspiratory muscle (lifts the first upper rib). When the ribs are fixed, it contracts on both sides and bends the cervical spinal column forwards. When contracted unilaterally, it flexes the same part of the spine and turns it to the left or right.

The posterior ladder muscle originates from the transverse processes of the 6th, 5th, 4th, and 3rd cervical vertebrae, moves downward behind the middle ladder muscle, and attaches to the outer surface of the second rib.

The posterior ladder muscle acts as an inspiratory muscle. When the ribs are stationary, it bends the cervical spine to the front (because it contracts on both sides). When contracted unilaterally, it flexes, turning the cervical spine to a certain side.

The long muscle of the neck occupies the entire anterolateral surface of the vertebral bodies, from the atlantus to the 3rd and 4th thoracic vertebrae. The middle sections of the muscle are slightly dilated. The length of muscle bundles varies, so the muscle is usually divided into three parts: upper oblique, medial-vertical, and lower oblique.

The long head muscle is located anterior to the long muscle of the neck. Its origin is the transverse processes of the 3rd to 6th cervical vertebrae. The place of attachment is the occipital bone (the muscle is located in front of the large occipital opening of this bone). The function of the long muscle is to tilt the head and flex the upper half of the cervical spine.

The anterior rectus abdominis muscle of the head is short. It starts where the lateral mass of the atlas and the anterior surface of the transverse process are located. From here, the muscle goes upwards and attaches to the bottom of the basilar part of the occipital bone, in front of the foramen magnum. The function of the muscle is to tilt the head to one side or the other (unilateral contraction) or to tilt the head forwards (bilateral contraction).

The origin of the lateral rectus abdominis muscle is the anterior part of the transverse process of the atlas. From here, the bundles run outwards and upwards. The muscle ends near the peri-maxillary process of the jugular process of the occipital bone. The function of the lateral rectus muscle depends on the type of contraction. In unilateral contraction, it tilts the head to the side, and in bilateral contraction, it tilts the head forwards.

Facial musculature

The facial muscles are closely intertwined and are located around the eyes, nose, ears, and mouth. The facial musculature includes mimic and masseter muscles that attach to the skin and soft tissues of the face. The overall structure includes about 20 flat skeletal muscles underlying the facial skin and scalp. All of them, with the exception of the cheek muscle, are not surrounded by fascia.

The facial muscles move the skin and soft tissues relative to the bony surface of the skull. This contributes to the formation of furrows, folds, wrinkles and dimples, which change facial expression and play a major role in matters of appearance. The mimic muscles are connected to the facial nerve (nervus facialis). When the facial nerve is damaged or inflamed, the corresponding muscles lose some or all of their function and do not work properly, resulting in visible changes in appearance (Fig. 14).

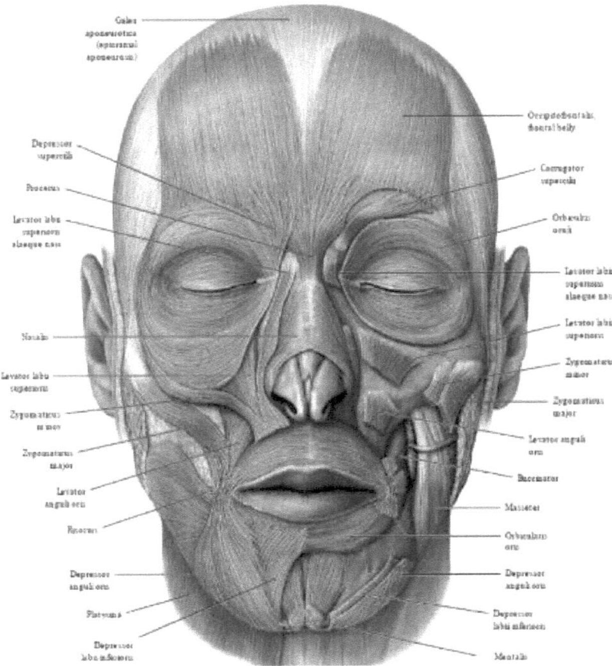

Figure 14: Facial mimic muscles

Most of the facial muscles contribute to the expression of emotions. The contraction of the muscles of this group results in changes in facial expression. Accordingly, the more frequently the mimic muscles are used, the more likely it is that premature wrinkles will appear on the face and neck, as the neck and facial muscles are closely linked. A distinctive feature is that the muscles in this group are relatively thin and attach directly to the skin, connecting with each other in separate bundles.

Muscles of the eye circumference

The circular muscle of the eye consists of several parts: ocular, eyelid, lacrimal. The orbicularis oculi muscle is responsible for the closure of the eye slit, the formation of folds in the eye socket and transverse wrinkles in the frontal area. The eyelid muscle is responsible for the closing of the eyelids. Lacrimal muscle - expansion of the lacrimal sac, filling with lacrimal fluid. Brow wrinkling muscle - responsible for the convergence of the eyebrow, takes part in the formation of interbrow folds. Pectoralis muscle - responsible for the middle part of the eyebrows and wrinkles the interbrow skin. Brow lowering muscle - lowers the eyebrow, contributes to the formation of transverse folds in the area of the nasal root (Fig. 15).

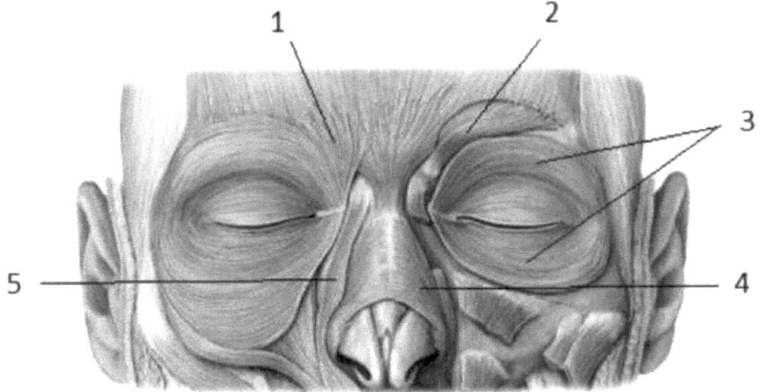

Figure 15: Muscles of the eye circumference: 1. Brow lowering muscle. 2. The muscle that wrinkles the eyebrow. 3. Oculomotor muscle. 4. Nasal muscle.

Muscles of the nasal circumference

The nasal muscle starts in the upper jaw, attaches to the nasal bone and is a group of muscles that consists of two parts. The outer one wraps around the wing of the nose, then widens slightly and at the midline and passes into a tendon. The inner part attaches to the posterior end of the cartilage of the nasal wing. The nasal muscle is responsible for the constriction of the nostrils. The nasal septal descending muscle is responsible for nostril dilatation at the entrance area (Fig. 15).

Muscles around the mouth

The muscles of the mouth belong to the cheek and lip group and represent a complex structural connection. The main functions are to control the movements of the lips and mouth. In total, there are 2 main categories of muscles in this group, which have different functional purpose: squeezing, raising and stretching the lips, lowering the corners of the mouth and others. The functions performed by the muscles of the mouth circumference correspond to the name (Fig.16):

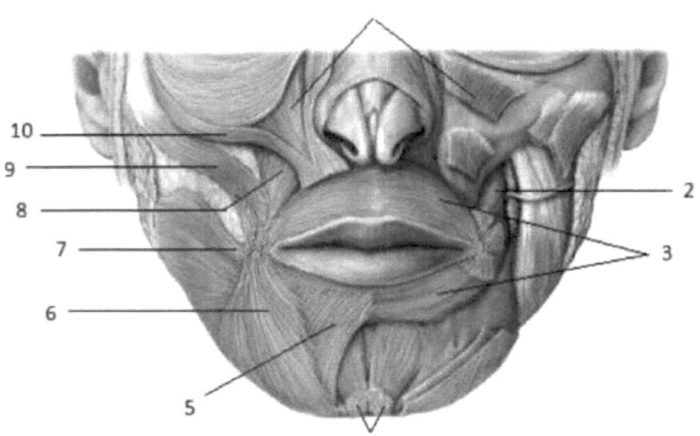

Figure 16: Muscles of the circumference of the mouth: 1. Raising the upper lip.
2. cheek muscle. 3. Circular muscle of the mouth. 4. Jawline muscle. 5. Lowering the lower lip. 6. The muscle that lowers the corner of the mouth. *7. The laughing muscle. 8. Lifting the corner of the mouth. 9. The large zygomatic muscle. 10. Small zygomatic.*

Chewing group of facial muscles

It ensures the process of mastication. It consists of *temporalis, masseter,* lateral and medial wing muscles. The temporal muscle is located in the temporal fossa. The lateral and medial wing muscles are located in the temporal fossa. The masseter muscle is located in the cheek area. The muscles of this group are attached to the lower jaw and are responsible for its movement in the temporomandibular joint when performing functions such as chewing and grinding (Figure 17).

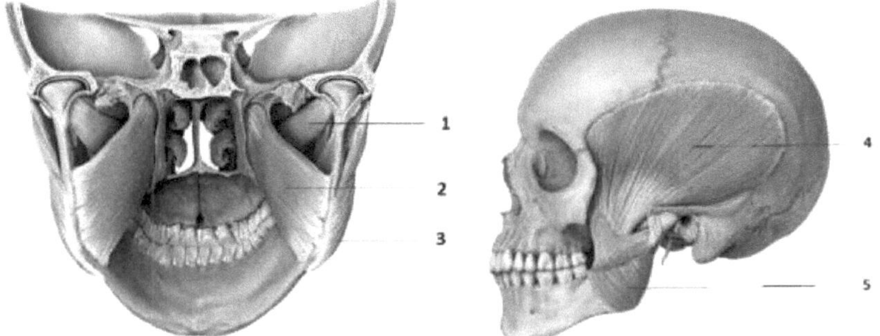

Figure 17. The masseter muscle: 1. Lateral wing muscle. 2. Medial wing muscle. 3. Chewing muscle. 4. Temporalis muscle. 5. Properly masseter muscle.

Langer lines

Langer lines - conventional lines on the skin surface indicating the direction of its maximum extensibility. They are named after a German anatomist who in 1861 studied in detail the elastic properties of human skin. They are round or ribbon-shaped, straight or twisted fibres of connective tissue of the skin. If their number increases in a certain place, they are connected to each other by branches in the form of a network, which is easily stretched in the direction of the fibres, and then regains its original form. Langer's studies have also shown that the plexus of connective tissue fibres is a lattice formation of vascular bundles with loops extending diagonally. The narrower the loops, the more parallel the vascular bundles. According to Langer, the direction of the course of elastic fibres of the skin is constant and varies in different areas of the body.

The strength properties of the skin depend on the direction of the acting force relative to the orientation of collagen fibres

(Langer lines). The maximum resistance of the skin is exerted when the direction of impact coincides with the orientation of these fibres, the specific tensile strength of the skin along the Langer lines requires a load almost 3 times greater than in the transverse direction.

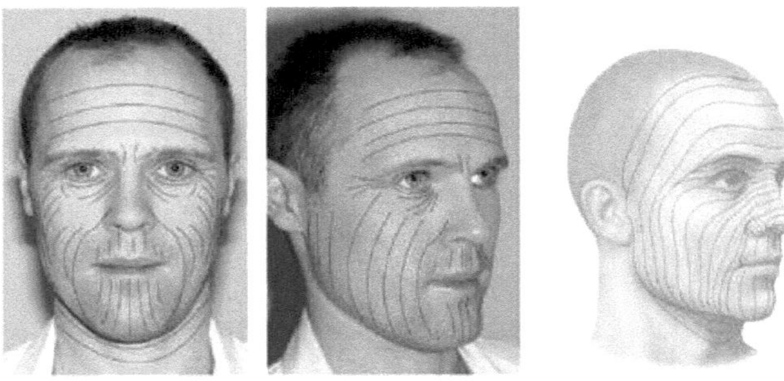

Figure 18: Langer lines on the facial skin surface

The shape of wounds in the skin, after removal of the wounding object, changes its shape. For example, wounds from the action of stabbing objects with a ribless surface are not round but slit-shaped, and their longitudinal dimensions in certain parts of the body are parallel. It is noted that there is no dependence of changes in the size of the skin preparation after exposure to fixing solutions in relation to the location of Langer lines.

PROBLEM RELEVANCE

Squamous cell carcinoma of head and neck organs is one of the common oncological pathologies and accounts for about 3% in the general morbidity structure of human malignant neoplasms [14,93]. The most frequent localisations (skin, oral cavity and oropharynx, nasal cavities, larynx, larynx) are characterised by a variety of clinical manifestations, difficulties in surgical treatment and high mortality rates [2, 9, 31, 27, 42, 74, 74, 80, 93, 104, 113, 117, 117, 123, 158, 158, 167].

Surgical treatment of head and neck tumours in most pathologies is the most radical and gives the best results.

Nevertheless, there are a number of issues that need to be solved. Thus, the main problem remains the formation of extensive postoperative defects that sharply disturb the main vital functions of the studied area and the appearance of patients [3, 24,91,157]. On the other hand, most surgeons sparingly spare the healthy tissues surrounding the tumour, reducing the volume of surgery, which is fraught with an increase in the number of recurrences [107].

The last decades are characterised by the development and introduction into oncological practice of methods of defect reconstruction with complex arterialised flaps on a pedicle with axial blood circulation, which allows expanding the indications for surgical treatment of locally advanced neoplasms. Nevertheless, this type of reconstruction has a number of disadvantages in addition to its advantages. Thus, the operation leads to rough scar deformations of donor sites, the percentage of purulent-necrotic complications remains quite high [126, 145], and the one-stage nature of the effect lengthens the time of the operation itself by 2-3 hours on average. Along with this, the mobility of all flaps on the pedicle is limited by the length of its pedicle, which requires the maximum proximity of the donor site to the place of plasty and the performance of additional incisions and, as a consequence, the formation of new scars on the head and neck. The use of thick musculoskeletal flaps, as the most viable ones, for plasty of oropharyngeal and laryngeal defects leads to narrowing of the lumen of the latter and impaired function [49].

Given the complex anatomo-functional features of the head and neck region, and the inherent consequences of PKROGSH treatment, as well as the wide range and combination of treatments that have specific implications on patients' quality of life (QOL), including physical, emotional, functional, social and occupational dysfunction, as well as the profound impact on families of PKROGSH patients [50, 160], which is significantly associated with overall survival [108, 141].

Depending on the location of the primary tumour, these patients experience specific symptoms during treatment, such as oral, swallowing and speech disorders, which often improve 6 months after treatment [26, 97]. However, long-term decline in quality of life in survivors with PKROGSH (at 10-year follow-up) is common [23]. Structured monitoring of patients' QoL in practice and clinical trials is important to provide individualised supportive care [120].

In the literature there are more and more frequent reports on the use of less massive dermofascial, mucofascial and musculoskeletal grafts cut from the adjacent areas of the operation. This tactic significantly reduces the operation time and gives the best cosmetic results without compromising the functions of the head and neck organs [3,15, 82, 109, 121].

Thus, the development of new leg flaps, the definition of clear indications for the use of traditional methods of plasty and the search for ways to reduce the number of purulent-necrotic complications is an urgent issue of modern oncology.

CHAPTER 1

RECONSTRUCTIVE AND RECONSTRUCTIVE SURGERIES AND QUALITY OF LIFE ISSUES IN PATIENTS WITH LOCALLY ADVANCED HEAD AND NECK CANCER (REVIEW)

In the general structure of oncological diseases, malignant neoplasms of the head and neck (HNNOSH) account for an average of 20-30% [8]. The annual incidence of head and neck cancer in the world ranges from 400,000 to 600,000 cases, with a mortality rate of about 223,000 to 300,000. The incidence ratio between men and women ranges from 2:1 to 4:1 [18, 93, 112, 167, 169].

Squamous cell cancer (SCC) accounts for about 90-95%, consistently ranking 6th among malignant tumours of the head and neck organs [66, 165] or 7% in the total incidence of human malignant neoplasms and is among the ten most common forms [8].

Despite the achievements of modern oncology, head and neck squamous cell cancer (HNSCC) consistently ranks 6th worldwide in the structure of mortality from malignant diseases [93, 80, 111, 162]. More than 50% of patients relapse within the first three years of diagnosis [18]. The overall 5-year survival rate for all localisations is still low and is as follows 51% in men and 61% in women [169].

Its association with smoking and alcohol consumption is well known [42, 128] but recently, especially in developed countries (USA, Canada, Europe, Japan, Australia), the incidence of oropharyngeal cancer associated with high-risk human papillomavirus (HPV) subtypes, mainly 16 and 18, has been increasing annually [27, 63, 87, 138, 139]. Tumour development is often correlated with younger age, better response to conservative chemoradiotherapy and better prognosis [27,80,95,139]. However, at this rate of growth, the annual incidence may surpass cervical cancer by 2020 [27,122,139].

According to WHO and the International Union Against Cancer (UICC), the number of head and neck cancer patients is steadily increasing annually, with an increasing percentage of patients with advanced stages of the disease [48], which, according to modern standards, necessitates multimodal combined and complex treatment methods, with surgery remaining the leading method [4,47,49,62,64, 102].

Despite the visual localisation, in most cases of PCROGSH in patients is often not diagnosed [29,38,42] until it reaches advanced stages (about 30% even in developed countries), requiring aggressive and expensive treatment that cannot be curative, and the probability of cancer recurrence in locally advanced forms reaches about 50% [34,59, 86].

It has been found that 50 to 80% of patients with OSA already have advanced stage III-IV cancers at the time of presentation [8, 9, 15, 18, 42, 66, 80]. Especially this "neglect phenomenon" is often observed in developing countries [76]. For example, according to Stephenson K.A, (2015) in a middle-income country like South Africa, 52% of patients requiring total laryngectomy initially required an emergency tracheostomy, indicating neglect. Consequently, treatment in such cases is mainly palliative [66, 132, 151, 1520].

Other reasons for late presentation are: uninformed and negligent attitude of patients to their own health condition, late presentation due to the absence of pain at the initial stages of the disease, which is the reason for patients' refusal of medical care, as well as ignorance of the initial symptoms of head and neck cancer, both by patients themselves and by general practitioners (dentists, family doctors, general practitioners, ENT doctors), lack of or limited access to medical services, lack of trust in doctors and, consequently, in the treatment of head and neck cancer.

Long waiting times for decision-making and treatment (surgery or radiotherapy) contribute to tumour progression. Patients often become inoperable while waiting for adequate treatment (surgery or radiotherapy); this complicates initial patient selection and treatment planning [114] confirmed that a one-month delay contributes to a 62% increase in tumour size and a 20% increase in new metastatic lymph nodes, consequently increasing the TNM score in 16% of patients studied; the mean time to tumour volume doubling was 3.13 months. In some institutions, to slow the progression of localised tumour

In advanced tumours, chemotherapy is used in an induction regimen [47,59]   (methotrexate or platinum-based drugs) while patients wait for definitive treatment, but there is no evidence that these modalities improve prognosis [110,122].

In early stages, treatment of head and neck squamous cell carcinoma is usually achieved with surgery or radiotherapy in 60 to 95% of cases (42,47,64,127). For locally advanced forms, treatment is usually comprehensive, and based on the histological characteristics of the tumour, combines either a combination of adjuvant chemotherapy, or chemoradiation therapy, followed by surgery, or chemoradiation therapy alone [122]. The treatment of recurrence depends on the localisation and histological characteristics of the tumour and the previous treatment and can be either palliative surgery or radiotherapy, or repeated chemoradiation therapy, and in cases where the tumour does not respond to palliative surgery and radiotherapy, chemotherapy remains [128, 132].

Surgical treatment of patients with locally advanced head and neck cancer in most localisations is the main and most radical method of treatment and gives the best results [24,36]. Despite the improvement of surgical and combined treatment methods over the last decade, there are still a number of problems that need to be solved [58]. Thus, the main problem remains the formation of extensive postoperative defects, which sharply disturb the basic vital functions of the studied area and the external (aesthetic) appearance of patients [3, 91, 157]. Accordingly, the majority of surgeons unnecessarily spare healthy tissues surrounding the tumour, reducing the volume of surgery, which is fraught with an increase in the number of recurrences [146].

expand the indications for surgical treatment of locally advanced neoplasms. Nevertheless, this type of reconstruction, in addition to its advantages, has a number of disadvantages [90, 150].

Thus, the operation leads to gross scar deformities of the donor sites, the percentage of purulent and necrotic complications remains quite high [49, 96, 140], and the one-stage nature of the effect lengthens the time of the operation itself by 2-3 hours on average. Along with this, the mobility of all flaps on the pedicle is limited by the length of its base, which requires the maximum proximity of the donor site to the place of plasty and additional incisions and, as a consequence, the formation of new scars on the head and neck. The use of complex musculoskeletal flaps, as the most viable ones, for plasty of oropharyngeal and laryngeal defects leads to narrowing of the lumen of the latter and impairment of their function [7, 154].

Due to the increasing morbidity rate and persistently extremely high mortality rate from locally advanced head and neck cancer [16], the search for optimal treatment tactics is considered an urgent task of modern clinical oncology [15, 85]. For specialists treating patients with this pathology, an extremely important issue is the choice of optimal treatment tactics, which will eliminate the tumour mass, improve the patient's quality of life and, in most cases, predetermine the prognosis of the disease [143, 144].

According to Osazuwa-Peters N. et al. (2018), in addition to high mortality rates from PCROGS, these patients have the second highest suicide rate after individuals with pancreatic cancer (63.4 vs. 86.4 cases per 100,000 population). Persistent psychological distress and reduced quality of life (QOL) are likely to be key factors underlying suicidality in patients with head and neck tumours [39, 50, 52, 67, 155].

Thus, an important aspect of this problem is the introduction of rehabilitation measures consisting in the application of reconstructive

plastic surgeries after tumour removal, effectively affecting the patients' quality of life [19, 86]. At the same time, the development of new stem flaps, the definition of clear indications for the use of traditional methods of plastic surgery and the search for ways to reduce the number of purulent-necrotic complications are urgent issues of modern oncology [60, 65, 85, 96, 140].

1.1 Evolution of reconstructive and reconstructive surgery

Whitaker I. S. et al. (2007) in his work entitled "The Birth of Plastic Surgery" [159] cites facts about Edwin Smith found in ancient Egypt in the work "Surgical Papyrus" dated to 3000 BC, which described the first in the history of mankind surgical treatment of mandibular and nasal fractures [61,72]. The treatment methods at that time were simple, such as repair of nasal bone fractures with subsequent sanation and tight tamponisation of the nostrils, with the application of a fixation dressing with splints.

In the 6th century BC, Sushruta of northern India described the first surgical procedures to repair a nasal defect by transferring a flap of skin from the forehead and cheeks. Sushruta's initial work in the pre-Christian era should have resulted in scant success, but based on the principle of "trial and error", the success of the "Indian flap" is so simple that the procedure is still used in modern reconstructive surgery [159].

The principles of defect reconstruction with pedicle flaps, which started by "trial and error" in pre-Christian history, were created and refined in the 19th century and became the fundamental basis for the impressive developments in the last decades of surgery. It is important to mention a few key moments in the development of tissue grafting during the 19th and 20th centuries: In 1829, Frick Hamburg published a book describing many alternative facial flaps. Soon after, Tripier, Malgaigne, Berrow, Estlander, von Grafe, Abbé, Denonvilliers, Rosenthal, Dieffenbach and Zeiss added new modifications and innovations in shifting tissue to adjacent areas within the face for reconstruction [83].

In the 1950s, the reconstruction of such defects moved to a new level and either a frontal or temporal flap combined with a split skin graft was used, but this method often resulted in gross scarring of the forehead skin or deformation of the temporal contours [125].

In 1958, Seidenberg et al. [149] described the successful use of the first revascularised flaps for one-stage reconstruction of a laryngopharyngeal defect of the cervical oesophagus with a segment of jejunum [147]. This event was indeed a milestone, but Seidenberg failed to translate his experience into a wide range of applications for many years, even in subsequent similar cases. His work gained popularity only when it was re-presented to the scientific community by Daniel and Taylor in 1973 [89].

The first work on experimental distant flap transplantation with microsurgical vascular anastomoses in dogs was published by R.

M. Goldwyn, D. L. Lamb and W. L. White (1963) [98, 153], and the first successful flap transplantation in humans was performed in September 1972. [100].

In 1965, Bakamjian first described the deltopectoral flap [84], Hence, some authors refer to McGregor in 1963 and Bakamjian in 1965 as pioneers who entered the modern era with the introduction of the first reliable axial circulation skin flap cut from the forehead and upper arm respectively. These flaps were used quite extensively by plastic surgeons to cover various kinds of defects from 1960 to 1970, but usually failed to duplicate the tissue defect. Others cite Buncke H.J. in microsurgical transplantation of the greater omentum to cover an extensive full-thickness scalp skin defect in 1972 [162].

One year later, in 1973, Daniel R.K. and Taylor G.L. reported the first successful transplantation of an autologous skin flap from the inguinal region to the sacral region using a surgical microscope, which was a divisive event in reconstructive surgery [89].

The first use of free skin flap in reconstructive and reconstructive head and neck surgery was in 1975 when Panje and Harashina simultaneously described the use of free flaps in tongue reconstruction [99, 129, 130].

The first successful reconstruction of the mandible was performed by Taylor in 1978, who used a free skin flap [89]. In this case, the inguinal flap was unable to retain the bone fragment of the *iliac* wing on the pedicle from the *superficial*

enveloping inguinal *artery* (*arteria circumflexa iliaca superficialis*). In his work, he showed that the blood supply of the iliac crest is provided by the branches of the deep iliac artery circumflexa iliaca superficialis
and can maintain nutrition to the skin over the bone. At that time, few head and neck surgeons were proficient in the technique of microsurgical flap harvesting.

In 1979, Ariyan S. described an arterialised musculocutaneous flap of the pectoralis major muscle, the discovery of which greatly expanded the possibilities of plastic surgeons [81]. In the following years, numerous researchers improved the technique of free flaps and expanded the indications for their use by opening perforant flaps (Koshima et al. 1989), using the peroneal flap to repair mandibular defects (Hidalgo D.A. 1989), reconstructing the tongue with a flap from *m. gracillis* (Yousif N.G. et al. 1999), using bioimplants in mandibular reconstruction (Moghadam H.G. 2001).

In 2005, the first partial face transplant was performed on Bernard Devauchelle in France. Later, in 2010, a complete face transplant was performed in Spain by Joan Pere Barret. Currently, for the block removal of locally advanced malignant tumours of the head and neck, the operation "face demasking" is used, which implies mask-like removal of the face with subsequent performance of an adequate volume of surgery and face replantation with preservation of the entire mimic function of the latter [109].

There is an opinion among the authors that it is impossible to talk about the advent of a "modern era" in reconstructive surgery until the majority of OSA oncologic surgeons become critically aware of the use of the wide range of available surgical reconstruction techniques.

Unlike other areas of the body, where aesthetic defects can

sometimes be covered by clothing or can even heal without serious complications by secondary tension, primary or early closure of defects of the head and neck is very important for several reasons. Firstly, preserving the integrity of the beginning of the digestive and respiratory tracts and consequently the patient's ability to eat and breathe are matters of paramount importance. Secondly, facial reconstruction is necessary for humans to socially communicate and socialise through facial expressions and facial expressions [91, 118]. Last but not least, covering the neurovascular bundles of the neck region to prevent aneurysms and arterial bleeding are challenges ahead for the oncological surgeon.

The choice of treatment tactics for locally advanced head and neck cancer is an extremely responsible and very complex task and must be developed by a multidisciplinary team of specialists, because it is on the correctness of this choice will depend on the further fate of the patient and the outcome of the disease.

When approaching reconstruction options for head and neck defects, a clear definition of the goals of reconstruction is an important element. Before proceeding to surgery, it is important to ask the question: "What type of reconstruction does the patient need?".

In 1982, Mathes and Nahai presented the so-called "reconstruction ladder" of defect closure from simple wounds to the most complex defects, which consists of 7 steps [148].

Many authors [148, 165, 166], when performing reconstructive surgeries, recommend adhering to the so-called "reconstruction ladder", consisting of several steps that define the step-by-step reconstruction of defects by: 1) Healing by secondary tension; 2) simple suturing of the wound edges; 3) plasty with skin flaps (split or full-layer); 4) tissue distraction method (expander dermotension   );   5) composite grafts; 7) displaced flaps; 8) flaps on a vascular pedicle; 9) free tissue complex transfer;   9) alloplastic materials or synthetic compounds: a) bioengineered, b) organ c) combined; such as porous polyethylene (Medpor), polytetrafluoroethylene (Gore-Tex), silicone and titanium, which are used for structural or bone reconstruction.

Today, this ladder has been supplemented with new "steps", i.e. such methods as negative pressure wound healing, the use of dermal matrices and reconstruction of defects with perforating flaps [112, 166].

As a rule, when planning individual defect reconstruction, the least difficult and safest step should be performed first, following the so-called "reconstruction ladder" while preserving form   and function.

With a full arsenal of reconstructive techniques, a head and neck surgeon should be able to answer the question "Which technique is best for a particular patient with a particular head and neck defect?".

The demands of modern plastic surgery in oncology dictate the need to obtain not only good functional but also to achieve good aesthetic results [97].

However, any scientific and clinical community that treats head and neck tumours is faced with the challenges of alternative multimodality treatment of head and neck squamous cell carcinoma (HNSCC), which include early and late complications, toxicity, limited functional and cosmetic outcomes, treatment plan failures, which in most cases dictate repeated palliative surgeries, still fraught with increased complications [49, 132, 140, 156].

In the late 19th and early 20th centuries, the main goal of surgeons - oncologists was ablative excision of locally disseminated head and neck tumours aimed at increasing the life expectancy of patients. In the USA even such a trend as "super-radicalism" appeared, which stipulated obligatory excision of all tissues affected by the tumour, including vital tissues, without taking into account the quality of life of patients and the conditions in which the patient fell after such an operation. Despite the fact that the survival rate of such patients did not change significantly for the better, this course has existed for several decades, and its supporters are still present today.

Rehabilitation of oncological patients, as a new direction in oncology, appeared in the middle of the last century. Its main thesis was partial or complete restoration of organ and organism functions as a result of surgical intervention and consists of functional, cosmetic and psychological rehabilitation of cancer patients.

Medical rehabilitation has two main goals: 1) selection of the most optimal surgical method of treatment that promotes maximum preservation of the anatomy and function of the organ. 2) determination of the complex of necessary therapeutic and reconstructive measures for optimal therapeutic effect and early recovery of patients' vital activity [1, 124].

In the clinical practice of oncology in recent years, sparing, organ-preserving operations are increasingly used, which, in turn, provide a sufficient level of radicality: various resection volumes - in laryngeal cancer up to stage III, parotidectomy with preservation of facial nerve branches - in parotid salivary gland cancer, tumour affecting one anatomical zone in the oral cavity. Unfortunately, such surgeries are unjustified in locally advanced cancer affecting more than one anatomical area of the head and neck, when in order to comply with the principles of ablative surgery it is necessary to perform a combined operation, including several organs in the volume of removed tissues [20]. Such a surgery volume is adequate and reduces the potential probability of locoregional tumour recurrence [33].

In case of extensive through tissue defects after radical removal of locally advanced tumours of the head and neck region, in the case of a full-thickness extensive defect of the cheek region, it is necessary to perform a two-layer reconstruction at the same time, i.e. to create a separate outer and inner wall, both in the skin area and from the inside, in the oral cavity. Individual publications describe the use of two distant flaps,   either from a twin free flap or from a double flap.

microsurgical flap; however, these extensive and prolonged surgical interventions are limited in elderly individuals due to somatic status and other objective reasons [53, 105, 119, 143].

We pointed out that oncological diagnosis and the proposed scope of surgical intervention in almost all patients are accompanied by the development of stress of varying severity. In the studies of a group of authors it was noted that the level of anxiety, stress and psychological discomfort in patients with PCRPSH is higher than in other cancer patients [50, 51, 67, 86, 165]. Studies have proved that pronounced psychogenic reactions have an undoubted influence on the frequency of postoperative complications [67, 86]. Prolonged hospital stay, feeding through a nasogastric tube, breathing through a tracheostomy, cosmetic facial disfigurements, severe disorders of vital body functions such as speech, chewing, swallowing, and breathing can lead to irreversible mental changes, up to suicidal outcomes [5]. As a result, all the efforts of doctors and the patient to eliminate a serious cancer will be absolutely useless, not to mention the financial aspect of the issue [92, 161].

The problem of rehabilitation and improvement of the quality of life of patients with head and neck tumours who have undergone radical surgery remains a complex issue that does not lose its relevance [1,7, 12,19, 23, 45,56, 124].

The issue of timely functional and cosmetic rehabilitation of oncological patients, which consists in planning and performing one-stage reconstructive and restorative surgeries for excision of locally advanced head and neck tumours [24, 37, 91], comes to the forefront. At the same time, the most reasonable approach is considered to be the one that allows adequate replacement of the tissue defect by means of a simple operation [54].

According to Zeynalova S.M. et al. (2016), the leading component of treatment of patients with locally advanced primary and recurrent head and neck cancer is surgical intervention with one-stage elimination of the postoperative defect with one of the types of plastic surgery [11].

The following types of extensive defects result from combined or extended combined operations for malignant tumours of the head and neck:

1) defects in skin, muscle and bone that do not communicate with cavities;

2) defects of mucous membranes, muscles and bones with preserved skin;

3) defects of mucous membranes, muscles and bones, but communicating with the skin surface over a large length;

4) through defects of the pharynx and larynx - pharyngostomies and laryngostomies [72].

Extensive tissue defects of the head and neck region cause severe functional and cosmetic disorders, which primarily impair important functions such as chewing, swallowing, breathing and speech [5,37, 71, 72].

In addition to functional disorders of the head and neck organs, the psychological state of patients is of great importance, to which doctors explain the necessary volume of tissues to be removed together with the tumour, including several adjacent anatomical areas, sometimes even organs. Such news is very hard to accept by patients, in particular when it comes to partial or complete loss of several vital functions of one or another organ. In addition, oncologists do not give any guarantees about the prognosis of treatment of malignant tumours (success of surgery, recurrence), which further aggravates the mental state of the patient. The necessity to apply a tracheostomy cannula, nasogastric tube to most of these patients, long tiring dressings and time spent in hospital, provision of more or less adequate, most often, tube feeding, which not every medical hospital is able to provide, - this is only a small part of the problems that need to be solved by the medical staff and the patient himself [66,86]. All of the above-mentioned problems cause more than 70% of patients to refuse surgery for locally advanced head and neck tumours and, as a result, condemn themselves to even more severe suffering and, ultimately, death.

More than 50% of locally advanced head and neck cancer cases develop recurrences, most of which are realised within 3 years after treatment [30, 31].

Among the malignant lesions of the larynx and larynopharynx, the share of squamous cell cancer is 90%. Already with locally advanced cancer 75-85% of patients come to treatment, 60-80% have regional metastases, in 50% of cases recurrences occur during the 1st year of follow-up, which is a poor prognostic factor. In stages I-II, the 5-year survival rate reaches 60%, in stages III-IV - 17-32% [33,68].

According to a number of authors, the mortality of patients with malignant neoplasms of the oral cavity in the first year after diagnosis was 34.8%-46.5% [12,13, 29,42,55].

Mortality of patients with locally advanced oropharyngeal cancer in the 1st year after treatment ranges from 30 to 40% [29,30]. The median survival of patients with recurrences realised within six months after chemotherapy with platinum-containing drugs in first or second line regimens does not exceed 6 months [31].

1.2 Quality of life of patients with head and neck tumours

Quality of life (QoL) issues for patients with malignant neoplasms (MN) are of critical importance. In 1999, the US National Cancer Institute and the American Society of Clinical Oncology determined that quality of life is the second most important quality of life indicator.

of significance as a criterion for assessing the results of antitumour therapy after survival - more important than the primary tumour response to treatment [108].

In studies, cure and survival rates were the highest treatment priorities for patients with PCROGS; however, parameters such as preservation of speech, reduction or absence of pain, and the ability to perform daily tasks were important to patients [114, 120].

At present, the available data on CV from clinical trials cannot be fully utilised for the benefit of patients individually   [40].

There is an emerging need to consider individualised approaches to assessing EF, which are of paramount importance in the treatment and monitoring of patients with SCIDD. In doing so, clinicians should consider the validity and appropriateness of methods for individualised assessment of EF, taking into account important aspects of the patient's life and priorities [114].

The quality of life of patients can be improved with the introduction of rehabilitation programmes, the aim of which is aimed at maximum restoration of physical, mental health, working capacity and social status of patients [39].

To date, there are many methods and tools to assess the impact of the disease, treatment methods and measurement of the parameters of QOL in patients with head and neck squamous cell cancer. In practice, 8 of them are mainly used, each of which reflects certain parameters of patients' health status [120]. There is no single gold standard for measuring the QOL in patients with SCSCC, but the European Organisation for Research and Treatment of Cancer (EORTC) questionnaires - EORTC QLQ-C30 and QLQ-H&N35 are the most widely used in the world literature [78]. Therefore, we used this methodology in our work.

Rehabilitation of oncology patients is a multistage process, the principles of which are early start of rehabilitation measures, dosage of load, continuity, consistency, complex and individual approach. Various specialists should be involved in the planning of rehabilitation measures: surgeon, radiation therapist, medical psychologist, prosthetist, speech therapist, oncologist-rehabilitation therapist [5, 19, 50, 51, 56, 86, 101, 120].

Partial or complete loss of speech, swallowing, chewing, and breathing disorders, which are severe consequences of surgical treatment of malignant tumours of the oropharyngeal zone and larynx [26, 134], determine the importance of speech rehabilitation [5, 19, 23, 43, 45, 56]. Rehabilitation measures can preserve and restore the functions of independent feeding, swallowing and speech in up to 92-97% of patients [5,26,69,].

According to Malagelada J. R. et al. (2015), swallowing disorders associated with both the presence of a volumetric mass and the results of its treatment accompany up to 65-70% of patients with head and neck tumours [168].

The possibilities of successful cure using surgical methods in

70-80% of patients with locally advanced oropharyngeal cancer are limited. Complete removal of the tongue with its root leads to persistent and severe disability of patients [12, 13, 66]. Speech function and swallowing are impaired or completely absent in these patients. Restoration of swallowing function can be achieved by restoring the motor function of preserved anatomical structures and mobility of transplanted tissues with adequately performed plasty [26, 66].

Thus, the issues of improving the quality of life in this contingent of patients is an urgent problem and consists in planning, developing and performing reconstructive and restorative surgeries aimed at restoring the lost functions of the head and neck organs and complex rehabilitation of patients [24].

Bachmann A.S. et al (2018) is of the opinion that little is known about the psychological constitution and potential adaptive mechanisms of these patients when they are admitted for inpatient treatment of patients with oral cancer. The aim of his study was to establish an acceptable research protocol and implement it to investigate patients' psychological responses at the initial stage of treatment in hospital [165].

Nelke K.H. et al. (2014) focusing on the quality of life of patients suffering from head and neck cancer note that their treatment often requires a multidisciplinary approach before and after surgery. Restoration of facial facial expression and aesthetics, articulation function, mastication and others often require long-term, compartmentalised rehabilitation. Quality of life is measured in the patient before and after surgery and complete treatment. The state of QL has different parameters depending on the patient's clinical diagnosis, type of treatment and surgery. It is also necessary to improve the patient's self-esteem and psychological evaluation [103].

Tripathi M. et al. (2015) describes the experience of 100 clinical cases of head and neck defect reconstruction in patients with stage 3-4 PCROGS with a flap on the pectoralis major muscle (MGM) in the period from 2006 to 2013. 86 patients had oral mucosa cancer, 8 patients had laryngeopharyngeal cancer, 3 patients had laryngeal cancer and 3 patients had salivary gland cancer. In 83% of cases the tumours had locally spreading character, which corresponded to T3-T4 symbols. In 95 patients the reconstruction was performed as a one-stage operation and in 5 patients with palliative purpose as a salvage operation. Using the BGM flap, mucosal defects were replaced in 84 patients, skin defects in 10 patients and combined defects in 6 patients. The percentage of complications was 40%, including partial necrosis of the flap - 10%, necrosis of the skin end parts - 30%, without a single case of total necrosis of the flap. Orostomies and pharyngostomies developed in 12 patients. In 10% of complicated cases repeated operations were necessary, complications in the form of pleural empyema developed in three patients. In conclusion, the authors note that, despite the fact that the "gold standard" of reconstructive surgery for head and neck tumours is free microsurgical flaps [131], the use of the latter is limited in a narrow circle of specialists, especially in developing countries, due to the high cost of the method and equipment and the lack of specialists [15, 73, 76, 88, 106, 151].

Anicin A. et al. (2015) [79] from the Department of Otorhinolaryngology of the Clinic of the Medical University of Ljubljana, Slovenia, analysed the oncological, functional and aesthetic results of head and neck defect reconstruction with the BGM flap in 39 patients with squamous cell cancer over 11 years (from 2001 to 2012). The age of the patients ranged from 40-76 years. A total of 40 flaps were used. The patients were divided into 2 groups: in the first group the treatment tactics initially started with surgery (n=19) 48.7%, and in the second group (n=20) 51.3% of patients with cancer recurrences underwent surgery and chemoradiotherapy, which had a palliative character. As a result, significantly better local control and recurrence-free survival rates were observed in the first group. Primary healing was noted in 32 patients, with a mean postoperative hospital stay of 22 days. Partial flap necrosis was noted in 3 cases. Both groups did not differ in functional and aesthetic results, speech intelligibility, impaired function of the upper limb and the flap's ability to close pharyngeal fistulas were almost identical. The authors concluded that due to its high viability, short engraftment time, low complication rate, and favourable aesthetic results in the donor sites in the majority of patients, the use of the BGM flap is an optimal material for primary plasty of defects in patients with head and neck cancer and in the so-called "salvage surgeries" [163].

With the constant improvement of systemic and local methods of treatment of oropharyngeal tumours, the survival rate of patients is steadily increasing, but after combined treatment they often have speech, chewing, swallowing, and breathing disorders, which significantly worsen the quality of life and make it difficult to

socio-psychological adaptation and integration

patients into society [141].

The study methodology, including time points of measurement and instrumentation, as well as the recruitment strategy, was also developed in three successive feasibility phases. The following qualitative (interview) and quantitative (questionnaires) criteria were used to assess patient responses: WOC-CA, brief COPE, HADS, EORTC QLQ C30-H&N35

and SAM/POMS. The results revealed that patients had high levels of anxiety and stress for whom a clear treatment strategy and tactics had not yet been developed. In addition, one third of the examined patients had severe levels of anxiety and depression, indicating a high vulnerability and propensy of this population to develop psychological disorders. Early in the treatment of oral cancer, potential psychosocial interventions should prioritise anxiety and depression so that patients can subsequently develop strategies to functionally adapt to these conditions [165].

Zhang X. et al. (2014) [75] analysed the effect of one-stage plasty of head and neck defects on quality of life (QOL), and in addition, comparing the differences between plasty with a BGM flap and a free flap from the anteroposterior surface of the thigh (ALTFF) in 110 patients. The IV version of the KJ questionnaire developed at the University of Washington was used to determine the parameters of KJ. The questionnaire was completed by 86 patients (78.2%) at least 24 months postoperatively. There were no differences in age, primary tumour size, disease stage and postoperative radiotherapy in the two groups. However, at follow-up, there were visible differences in both groups in sex, shorter operation time and complication rate. A comparative analysis was performed to compare the differences in QOL between patients reconstructed with the BGM flap and ALTFF. Patients in the free flap group had fewer complications in shoulder function, but speech function was worse than patients in the stem flap group. The results of this study provide useful information for physicians and patients when discussing treatments for head and neck cancer.

Rehabilitation of patients with OHSS is accepted as an integral part of patient care, aiming to improving and maximising the patient's quality of life. Patients who have undergone extended surgery for head and neck tumours face many challenges and require a specific rehabilitation programme. This review collates evidence specific to head and neck cancer patients and divides the programme into five domains : functional, medical, aesthetic, psychological and social. This provides a common framework for addressing these unique rehabilitation requirements (124).

According to Sammut L. et al. (2014) [147] head and neck cancer and its treatment leads to a significant reduction in quality of life and presents problems for both patients and their relatives and carers. Physical activity has been found to be particularly important in counteracting symptoms that reduce QoL, including depression, fatigue, anxiety and restlessness.

Bannister M. et al. (2015) reviewed in detail 13 articles on rehabilitation after laryngectomy, cervical dissections, major surgical volumes in OGS and microvascular reconstruction. Articles on general preoperative preparation and postoperative care were also reviewed. After conducting a systematic review and reviewing the literature on enhanced rehabilitation programmes in the surgical treatment of head and neck tumours, we concluded that there is considerable evidence to support the feasibility of enhanced rehabilitation interventions in head and neck surgery that can benefit patients and that surgeons should be aware of [85].

To evaluate the role of regional and free tissue transfer for palliative treatment of head and neck cancer involving large areas of skin, the authors [132] conducted a retrospective review of patients who received

treatment of head and neck cancer with skin involvement at Mount Sinai Medical Centre over a 5-year period (2006-2010). Only patients with extensive skin involvement and inoperable

tumours who underwent palliative tumour resection with one-stage reconstruction were included in the review. Results: 25 patients fulfilled the inclusion criteria for the review. Of these, 14 patients (56%) underwent reconstruction of defects with pedicled flaps and 11 patients (44%) underwent reconstruction with free microsurgical flaps,   19 patients (76%)
received adjuvant palliative radiotherapy and/or chemotherapy. Four patients (16%) had distant metastases at the time of surgery, and the median time to develop distant metastases after surgery was 6 months. Median survival was 9.5 months. Conclusions: palliative surgery with reconstruction is a reasonable treatment option for patients with inoperable tumours with extensive skin involvement. These do not improve survival, but the elimination of odour, bleeding, intolerable pain and infection associated with skin involvement can improve the patient's quality of life.

Patel K. et al (2014) note that rehabilitation, functional outcomes and acceptable quality of life are the main goals of oral reconstructive surgery, even in advanced stages where survival is limited. The authors report the functional plastic results observed in glossectomies in which reconstruction was performed using three different techniques. A total of 264 flaps were used, which the authors divided into three groups of 15 patients. The groups were divided as follows: 1) free forearm flap, 2) large pectoralis muscle flap; 3) nasolabial flap. All groups had an extremely low rate of complete flap necrosis, but complications in the form of fistulas and orostomies were significantly frequent in the musculocutaneous flap group. There were good results in the recovery of speech and swallowing function in the majority of patients. In less than 15% of the patients, incomprehensible speech and the need for constant wearing of a nasogastric tube for feeding were noted.

The BGM flap showed its best functional characteristics in total and subtotal glossectomy with excision of the muscles of the floor of the mouth. The free forearm flap proved to be reliable and safe with its lower thickness and flexibility, especially after partial glossectomy. The nasolabial flap was confirmed to be the flap of choice for partial resections of the tongue and anterolateral portions of the floor of the mouth. To summarise, the author notes that free flaps do not replace conventional musculoskeletal flaps, but they are an ideal alternative for specific and selected indications [133].

Studies have shown that measurement of QOL parameters can help predict survival [Aarstad H.J. et al., 2014]. In a recent study, the baseline level of QOL was a prognostic indicator of overall observed survival in head and neck cancer patients and was used to stratify patients in clinical trials [Urba S. et al., 2012]. These findings highlight the importance of assessing the patient as an individual rather than simply treating their disease, however, meaningful global data on CV in SCCHD are still scarce [92], so it is important to understand how to better and effectively assess CV in patients with SCCHD so that treatment and support interventions can be tailored to the needs and outcomes of patients individually.

Wolff K.D. et al. (2015), giving a brief overview of the development and current clinical application of perforator flaps, states that the discovery of these flaps is a sign of significant progress in the surgical reconstruction of head and neck defects, but whether they are the next step up the "reconstructive ladder" is still unknown. As an example, the author cites 4 flaps from the lower limb that he used to close oral defects. But when one considers the range of new donor sites and the precision of flap design offered by perforator flaps, it becomes apparent that the potential of this new technique, has not yet been reached

[166].

To answer the question: "Is advanced age a contraindication to surgical treatment of patients with head and neck cancer?". (Yang R. et al., 2014) [105] conducted a retrospective analysis and detailed review of the histories of 53 patients aged 80 years and older (mean age 85 years) who underwent surgical treatment for head and neck malignancies between 1996 and 2011. The average duration of follow-up was 32 months. The most common comorbidity was cardiovascular disease (43%). Squamous cell cancer of the oral cavity and oropharynx was verified in 45 patients (85%). The operations performed included 40 neck dissections and 12 microvascular free flaps. The mean hospitalisation period was 6.4 days. The increase in hospitalisation period was significant in patients who underwent grafting with free flaps (p < 0.01). There were no cases of perioperative death or flap necrosis. 34 (61.4%) patients were discharged in a

The most common postoperative complications were cardiovascular complications (n = 8). The most frequent postoperative complications were cardiovascular (n = 8), infectious complications (n = 10), and delirium (n = 6). Reconstruction with a free flap had no adverse effect on the period of hospitalisation in the hospital (p > 0.05). More than 75% of patients did not experience any serious limitations in daily life. Extended surgery for malignant head and neck tumours can be tolerated in elderly patients using careful patient selection. Age alone should not be a major factor in the treatment of patients with head and neck cancer [105].

As the incidence of head and neck cancer in the elderly increases, their treatment often requires a multidisciplinary approach, which can be quite painful. Elderly patients (in this case, designated as over 65 years of age) with HNC often have significant comorbidities and impaired overall functional status, which can interfere with their ability to accept and tolerate combined treatment. Therefore, they have often been excluded from clinical trials that have defined standards of care. Therefore, adapting cancer therapies for elderly patients with OHSS can be quite challenging. In this article, a comprehensive literature review was conducted to better understand and discuss issues regarding therapeutic recommendations that are specific to patients 65 years of age and older. Evidence suggests that elderly patients have similar survival outcomes compared to their younger counterparts, but may have a worse tolerance to toxicity, especially when treatment is intensified. Consequently, older patients need more support throughout the treatment process. Studies incorporating geriatric tools are needed, potentially improving patient selection and tolerance to intensive treatment [164].

Thus, the analysis of available scientific studies on the problem concerning surgical aspects of head and neck squamous cell carcinoma treatment, questions about postoperative complications, defect elimination, restoration of lost functions and, affecting significantly on the QOL, predetermine the need for further study and development of this problem.

CHAPTER 2

CHARACTERISATION OF OWN CLINICAL MATERIAL

2.1 General characteristics of clinical observations

Our study was based on clinical observations of 169 patients with squamous cell carcinoma of the head and neck region aged 25 to 92 years who received treatment in the department of general oncology of the State Institution "Republican Oncological Scientific Centre" of the Ministry of Health and Social Protection of the Population of the Republic of Tajikistan during the period from 2008 to 2019. The main criterion for the sample of patients was the presence of histologically verified cancer of the head and neck organs. Of these, 151 (89.3%) patients had locally advanced tumour process and corresponded to stages III - IVA, IVB. All patients received combined and complex treatment according to the treatment standards accepted in the country, with a mandatory stage of surgical removal of the tumour.

To compare the treatment results, all patients were divided into 2 groups. The main criterion for dividing the patients into the studied groups was the difference in the volumes of operative intervention   , i.e., the difference in the volume of the intervention performed.

reconstructive-restorative stage of surgical intervention.

The main group included 108 (63.9%) patients who, after removal of the primary tumour and dissection of the lymphogenic metastasis pathways, underwent one-stage reconstruction of the formed defects with flaps with axial blood supply.

one-stage reconstruction of the formed defects with flaps with axial blood supply was performed.

The control group included 61 (36.1%) patients who underwent tumour excision with replacement of the resulting tissue defect with either free skin graft (or autologous skin) or local tissues, and sometimes without plasty. Our study is a parallel prospective-retrospective study. From the total cohort (n = 169) 102 (60,4%) patients were treated prospectively, and 67 (39,6%) - retrospectively, and the proportion of prospective patients in the main group was 59,3% (64 patients), and in the control group - 62,2% (38 patients). The criteria for exclusion of patients were their refusal of surgical intervention, presence of severe intercurrent somatic pathology, psychiatric diseases, and disagreement to participate in the study. This study was approved by the ethical committee of the Abuali ibn Sino State Medical University in accordance with the provisions of the Helsinki Declaration of the World Medical Association of the latest revision. The study design is presented in Figure 19.

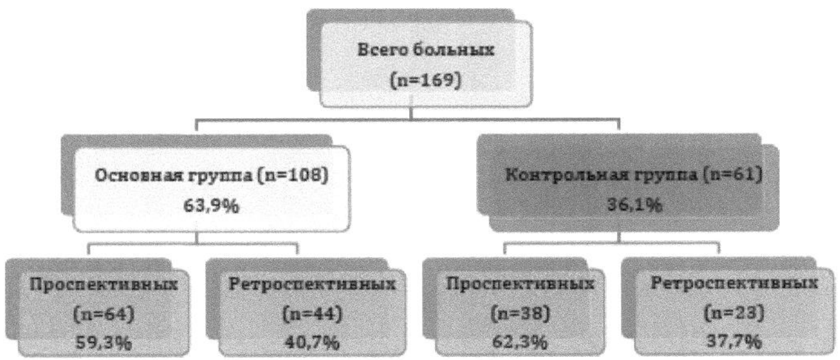

Figure 19. - Study design

The study included 169 patients aged 25 to 92 years. Of them, men were - 107 (63.3%), women - 62 (36.7%). The mean age of the patients was 61.0 years, the mean age of men was 60.6 and of women - 61.8 years (Table 1).

Table 1. - Distribution of patients by sex and age

Age	Men		Women		Number of patients				p
					n absolute number		в %		
	OG	KG	OG	KG	OG	KG	OG	KG	
25 - 44	8	6	4	1	12	7	11,1	11,5	0,856
45 - 59	22	16	12	9	34	25	31,5	41,0	0,214
60 - 74	23	13	18	9	41	22	38,0	36,0	0,807
75 - 90	12	4	7	1	19	5	17,6	8,2	0,093
over 90	1	2	1	0	2	2	1,8	3,3	0,558
Total:	66 (61,1)	41 (67,2)	42 (38,8)	20 (32,2)	108	61	100%	100%	

Note: OG - main group, CG - control group. *p* - statistical significance of the difference between the indicators of the main and control groups (%² Pearson).

As can be seen from Table 1, among the patients included in the study, both in the main and control groups, there was a significant predominance of men over women, with a ratio of 2:1 - in the main group 66 (61.1%) versus 42 (38.9%), in the control group - 41 (67.2%) versus 20 (32.8%). The peak of morbidity in both groups was observed in the age groups 45-59 and 60-74 years, in the main group - 75 (69.5%) and in the control group - 47 (77%), i.e. middle-aged and elderly people prevailed. It should be noted that with age patients develop various comorbidities accompanying oncological diseases: cardiovascular diseases, diabetes mellitus, diseases of respiratory system, urinary system, which often require conservative treatment and sometimes complicate the treatment of patients, in particular, planning and carrying out combined and extended-combination treatment.

surgical interventions, as well as aggravating negatively affect the rehabilitation of patients in the postoperative period (Table

2).

Table 2. - Presence of comorbidities in the studied groups of patients

Associated disease	Main group, n = 108	Control group, n = 61	*P*
Gastrointestinal systems	83 (76,8%)	47 (77,0%)	0,977
Urinary system	71 (65,7%)	36 (59,0%)	0.320
Cardiovascular system	54 (50,0%)	24 (39,3%)	0.183
Anaemia of varying degrees	34 (31,4%)	21 (34,4%)	0.695
Reproductive system	17 (15,7%)	17 (27,8%)	0.059
Endocrine system	15 (13,8%)	3 (5,0%)	0.120
Viral hepatitis B and C	12 (11,1%)	5 (8,2%)	0.546

Note: p - statistical significance of the difference between the indicators of the main and control groups (by Pearson's %2 criterion).

As can be seen from Table 2, the most frequent comorbidities in both the main and control groups were: pathology of the gastrointestinal tract in the form of cholecystitis and pancreatitis (76.8% vs. 77.0%), inflammatory diseases of the kidneys and urinary tract (pyelonephritis, urolithiasis) - (65.7% and 59.0%), cardiovascular system in the form of arterial hypertension of various degrees and risks, atherosclerosis of the aorta and cerebral vessels (50.0% and 39.3%), blood system, anaemia of varying severity (31.4% and 34.4%), reproductive system (chronic endometritis in women, prostatitis in men (15.7% and 27.8%), endocrine system (type II diabetes mellitus, diffuse goiter of varying degrees) 13.8% and 5.0%, and various infectious and allergic diseases (viral hepatitis B, C, polyvalent allergy) 11.1% and 8.2%. Consequently, the age of patients and their initial somatic safety is an important factor in decision making and development of treatment tactics for this category of patients.

The presence of concomitant genitourinary infectious pathology in a significant proportion of patients gives us reason to assume an infectious etiology of head and neck cancer, in particular human papillomavirus (HPV), strains of high oncogenicity, which requires further research in this direction.

All operations were performed under general endotracheal anaesthesia using neuroleptanalgesia and ketamine drugs. To achieve sedation, improve the course of anaesthesia, relieve psycho-emotional stress and reduce hypersalivation, all patients were premedicated 45 minutes before intubation with intramuscular injection of 1% p/r analgin 2.0, 1% p/r dimedrol 1.0, and 1% p/r atropine sulphate 1.0. In addition, the patients were given sedatives before and on the day of surgery.

In the presence of pain syndrome, guided by its severity, adequate analgesia with non-narcotic and narcotic drugs was performed using an analgesia protocol.

One of the significant prognostic factors in the treatment of head and neck squamous cell carcinoma is the stage of the disease or the degree of spread of the tumour process. The studied groups included mainly patients with locally advanced tumour process, as this cohort of patients is the most difficult to treat and even if their treatment is successful, their quality of life suffers to a varying degree. The localisation of the primary tumour in the studied groups is shown in Table 3.

Table 3. - Distribution of patients by sex and primary tumour location

	Paul		Main group	Control group	Total %, (n)		$R\,x^2$
	H us	Wi fe.					
Skin coverings	25	11	24 (22,2%)	12 (19,7%)	21,3%	(36)	0,698
Alveolar process of the mandible	25	11	25 (23,1%)	11 (18,0%)	21,3%	(36)	0,436
Cheek mucosa	13	12	23 (21,3%)	2 (3,3%)	14,7%	(25)	0,004
Language	13	10	7 (6,5%)	16 (26,2%)	13,6%	(23)	<0,001
Red lip line	10	5	14 (13,0%)	1 (1,6%)	8,8%	(15)	0,028
Upper jaw	8	6	1 (0,9%)	13 (21,3%)	8,2%	(14)	<0,001
The floor of the	9	2	9 (8,3%)	2 (3,3%)	6,5%	(11)	0,340

mouth							
Alveolar process of the maxilla	2	4	2 (1,9%)	4 (6,6%)	3,5%	(6)	0,113
Larynx	2	-	2 (1,9%)	-	1,1%	(2)	-
Thyroid gland	0	1	1 (0,9%)	-	0,5%	(1)	-
Total:	10	7	62	(3)	108 (100%)	61 (100%)	100%	169

Note: this localisation is covered in a separate Table 4.

p - statistical significance of the difference between the indicators of the main and control groups (by Pearson's $\%^2$ criterion).

The data shown in Table 3 indicate that the most frequent tumour localisations were: the skin of the head and neck and the alveolar process of the mandible 21.3% each, the cheek mucosa 14.7%, and the tongue 13.6%. In other words, the oral cavity, occupying a central position, is the area from which up to 4050% of head and neck tumours originate. The red lip border, the upper jaw, and the mucosa of the floor of the oral cavity occupied an intermediate position in terms of frequency. Among the least rare localisations were cancer of the mucosa of the alveolar process of the maxilla (3.5%), cancer of the larynx (1.1%), and thyroid cancer (0.5%).

When analysing the patients according to the study groups, it can be seen that in the main group, the tumour was most often located in the region of the alveolar process of the mandible, head and neck skin and cheek mucosa in almost equal numbers 25 (23.1%), 24 (22.2%), 23 (21.3%) cases respectively. Relatively less frequently the tumour was localised on the red border of lips - in 14 (13,0%) patients, mucosa of the floor of the mouth - 9 (8,3%), tongue - 7 (6,5%). Cancer of the mucosa of the alveolar process of the upper jaw and larynx was observed with the same frequency in 2 (1,9%) cases, also in the lowest frequency the tumour was localised in the upper jaw and thyroid gland - 1 case each, which made up (0,9%) of the total cohort of patients.

In the control group, the most frequent localisations of

malignant tumours were the tongue - 16 (26.2%), the upper jaw - 13 (21.3%), the skin of the head and neck - 12 (19.7%) and the alveolar process of the lower jaw - 11 (18.0%), which together amounted to 85.2%. Less frequently, the tumour was located on the mucosa of the alveolar process of the upper jaw - 4 (6.6%), the mucosa of the floor of the mouth and cheek - 2 (3.3%) cases each, and the red border of the lower lip - 1 (1.6%) case. It is worth emphasising that in our study, the frequency of patients with tongue and maxillary cancer who did not undergo defect plasty is relatively high in the control group. This discordance in the frequency of tumour occurrence in the control group in relation to the main group is probably due to the fact that in tongue and maxillary jaw cancer, free microsurgical grafts (radial flap from the forearm, trapezoidal flap) are more acceptable and optimal materials for defect reconstruction [142], which we do not use due to the inadequacy of the technique.

Based on the examination data, each patient was individually justified the treatment algorithm and reconstruction method. At the stage of surgery planning, flap marking was performed according to standard anatomical landmarks, as well as to assess the state of the donor area vessels using ultrasound Doppler ultrasonography.

The main objective of reconstructive surgery is to replace one or more epithelial surfaces with a flap, and in some cases to fill the deficit of the underlying non-epithelial tissues. On this basis, we consider it rational to divide patients depending on the characteristics of tissues (skin or mucosal epithelium) from which the tumour developed into two large groups - mucous membranes (group 1) and skin (group 2).

Based on Table 4, in the total cohort of patients in the majority of cases, cancer localised on the mucous membrane of the oral cavity was found in 101 (59.8%) cases. This is explained by the fact that the oral cavity, being the beginning of the digestive system, is often exposed to carcinogenic chemical factors such as smoking, use of tobacco products - nasvay, alcoholic beverages, as well as mechanical stimuli - from caries to improperly fitted dentures.

Thus, in the main group the proportion of this contingent of patients was 61.1%, and in the control group - 57.4%, i.e. almost the same frequency of occurrence. Cancer of the upper jaw was observed in 14 patients (8.3%), of which 1 patient was in the main group and 13 patients in the control group, which accounted for 0.9% and 21.3%, respectively. Laryngeal cancer and thyroid cancer occurred in relatively low frequencies of 2 and 1 observations, respectively, only in the main group, and there were no patients with this localisation in the control group.

Lip cancer, according to the TNM tumour classification system, is considered together with the oral cavity and occupies an intermediate position between the skin and mucous membranes. Consequently, we included this localisation in group 1, which comprised 15 observations (8.9%), of which the majority - 14 (12.9%) patients were in the main group and 1 (1.6%) patient in the control group.

Of the total cohort (n = 169), we observed head and neck skin tumour lesions in 36 (21.3%) cases, of which the proportion of patients in the main group was 24 (14.2%) cases and 12 (6.1%) in the control group (Table 4).

Table 4. - Distribution of patients according to tumour localisation on the skin (n=36)

Tumour localisation	Core group	Control group	Total n, (%)	P
Cheekbone region	3	3	14 (38,9%)	0,137

Nose	5	-		
Cheek	2	-		
Forehead	-	1		
Auricle	5	3		
Parotid region	3	-	11 (30,5%)	0,191
Temporal area	5	2		
Dark region	1	2	10 (27,8%)	0,734
Neck	-	1	1 (2,8%)	-
Total	**24**	**12**	**36**	**0.698**

Note: p - statistical significance of the difference between the indicators of the main and control group (by the criterion $\%^2$ Pearson).

The most frequent (Table 4) skin cancers of the zygomatic region, nose, cheek and forehead were 14 (38.9%), whereas skin cancers of the auricle, parotid region and temporoparietal region occurred in almost equal frequencies in 11 (30.5%) and 10 (27.8%) observations, respectively. The lowest frequency of skin lesions on the posterior surface of the neck was 1 (2.8%) case.

The staging of the tumour process depending on the extent of the primary tumour was performed according to the TNM International Classification of 2018 (8th edition), which is up to date [77].

The distribution of patients according to the size of the primary tumour was as follows: in the main group, in 14 (12.9%) patients the tumour corresponded to the T2 symbol, in 31 patients (28.7%) - to the T3 symbol, and in 63 (58.3%) patients it corresponded to the T4 symbol. The low rate of relatively early stage of the disease (T2) (12.9%), especially in mucosal cancer of the alveolar process of the mandible, tongue cancer, mucosal cancer of the floor of the oral cavity and alveolar process of the maxilla, is noteworthy (Table 5).

Table 5. - Distribution of patients in the main and control

groups by localisation and spreading
<u>**primary tumour**</u>

Tumour localisation		T2 %, (n)	T3 %, (n)	T4 %, (n)	Total %, (n)
Alveolar process of the mandible	OG	0,9 (1)	2,8 (3)	19,4 (21)	23,1 (25)
	KG	-	1,6 (1)	16,4 (10)	18,0 (11)
	P	-	0,953	0,623	0,436
Face, head and neck skin	OG	2,7 (3)	5,5 (6)	13,9 (15)	22,1 (24)
	kg	1,6 (1)	4,9 (3)	13,1 (8)	19,7 (12)
	P	0,953	0,858	0,927	0,698
Cheek mucosa	OG	1,9 (2)	10,2 (11)	9,3 (10)	21,4 (23)
	KG	1,6 (1)	1,6 (1)	-	3,3 (2)
	P	0,613	0,078	-	0,002
Red lip line	OG	4,6 (5)	4,6 (5)	3,7 (4)	12,9 (14)
	kg	-	-	1,6 (1)	1,6 (1)
	P	-	-	0.774	0,028
Language	OG	0,9 (1)	2,8 (3)	2,8 (3)	6,5 (7)
	kg	8,2 (5)	13,1 (8)	4,9 (3)	26,2 (16)
	P	0,044	0,022	0,773	<0,001
The floor of the mouth	OG	-	2,8 (3)	5,6 (6)	8,4 (9)
	kg	-	1,6 (1)	1,6 (1)	3,3 (2)
	P		0,953	0,410	0,340
Alveolar process of the maxilla	OG	-	-	1,9 (2)	1,9 (2)
	kg	-	-	6,6 (4)	6,6 (4)
	p			0,249	0,249
Upper jaw	OG	-	-	0,9 (1)	0,9 (1)
	kg	1,6 (1)	3,3 (2)	16,4 (10)	21,3 (13)
	P	-	-	<0,001	<0,001
Larynx	OG	1,9 (2)	- -	-	1,9 (2)
	kg	-	-	-	0
Thyroid gland	OG	-	-	0,9 (1)	0,9 (1)
	kg	-	-	-	0
Total	OG	12,9% (14)	28,7% (31)	58,3% (63)	100% (108)
	kg	13,1% (8)	26,2% (16)	60,7% (37)	100% (61)
	P	0.834	<0,001	0.768	

Note: p - statistical significance of the difference between the indicators of the main and control groups (by Pearson's $\%^2$ criterion).

The control group showed almost the same pattern of stage distribution (Table 6).

Table 6. - Degree of tumour spread depending on the localisation in the main and control groups

Stage / Localisation^ / Tumours		II		III			IVA, IVB				Total, absolute number, (%)	P
Face, head and neck skin	OG	3	-	5	1	-	12	2	1	-	24 (22,2%)	0,698
	KG	2	-	2	1	-	6	1	-	-	12 (19,7%)	
Alveolar process of the mandible	OG	1	-	2	1	-	7	10	3	1	25 (23,1%)	0,463
	kg	-	-	-	1	-	2	5	3	-	11 (18,0%)	
Cheek mucosa	OG	2	-	3	7	1	5	4	1	-	23 (21,3%)	0,004
	kg	1	-	1	-	-	-	-	-	-	2 (3,3%)	
Red lip line	OG	4	-	3	2	-	3	1	-	1	14 (13,0%)	0,028
	kg	-	-	-	-	-	-	1	-	-	1 (1,6%)	
The floor of the mouth	OG	-	-	1	2	-	1	3	1	1	9 (8,3%)	0,340
	kg	-	-	-	-	1	1	-	-	-	2 (3,3%)	
Language	OG	1	-	1	-	2	1	-	2	-	7 (6,5%)	<0,001
	kg	5	-	4	3	1	-	1	2	-	16 (26,2%)	
Alveolar process of the upper jaw	OG	-	-	-	-	-	1	1	-	-	2 (1,9%)	0,249
	kg	-	-	-	-	-	4	-	-	-	4 (6,6%)	
Upper jaw	OG	-	-	-	-	-	1	-	-	-	1 (0,9%)	<0,001
	KG	-	-	2	-		10	-	-	1	13 (21,3%)	
Larynx	OG	2	-	-	-	-	-	-	-	-	2 (1,9%)	-
Thyroid gland	OG	-	-	-	-	-	1	-	-	-	1 (0,9%)	-
Total:	OG	13	0	15	13	3	32	21	8	3	108 (100%)	
	kg	8	0	9	5	2	23	8	5	1	61 (100%)	
	p	0,071		0,941	0,605	0,349	0,282	0,409	0,08	0,959		

Note: OG - main group, CG - control group. p - statistical significance of the difference between the indicators of the main and control groups (by Pearson's u2 criterion)

Thus, 8   (13.1%) patients had   tumour stage corresponded to the T2 symbol, in 16 (26.2%) patients - to the T3 stage, and in 37 (60.7%) patients - to the T4 symbol. It should be emphasised that in the main and control groups in the absolute majority of cases - 87% and 86.9%, respectively - there was a locally advanced tumour process. In order to compare the initial parameters of the patients' tumour process and to obtain the most approximate results we decided to study in detail the interrelation of the tumour process spreading from its localization. It follows from the data of Table 6 that 69 patients (78,8%) from the total cohort of patients - 48 (44,4%) in the main group and 21 (34,4%) in the control group - along with locally spread tumour process were diagnosed with clinically enlarged regional lymph nodes of the neck, which were verified by cytomorphological examination. For this purpose, we used the technique
fine-needle aspiration biopsy (puncture) of the affected lymph node(s) (including under the control of an ultrasound transducer). These patients came for treatment already with metastatic lesions of regional lymph nodes and only in 2 (1,1%) patients metastatic lesions of mediastinal lymph nodes (M1) were revealed during treatment. In these cases, the tumour process is considered locally advanced based on the size of the primary tumour, and the presence of metastatic regional lymph nodes, according to the results of numerous publications, significantly worsens the prognosis of the disease, reducing the 5-year survival rate by 50% [76].
The largest number of observed patients in the main and control groups were treated for cancer corresponding to stage IV

grading (T - $N_{341\text{-}20}$) M- 106 (62.7%) cases. In the main group, this contingent comprised 67(62.0%) patients and in the control group, 39 (63.9%) patients. In 166 (98.2%) patients the tumour was represented by squamous cell cancer (Table 7).

Table 7. - Morphological verification of tumours

Histological type of tumour	Number of observations	%
Squamous cell cancer with keratinisation	101	59,7%
Squamous cell cancer without keratinisation	65	38,4%
Adenocarcinoma of the salivary gland	1	
Follicular carcinoma of the thyroid gland	1	1,77%
Ameloblastic carcinoma	1	

Of these, 101 (59.7%) had squamous cell keratinising cancer and 65 (38.4%) had squamous cell cancer without keratinisation. In the remaining 3 patients (1.77%) the tumours morphologically represented parotid adenocarcinoma.

salivary gland, follicular thyroid carcinoma and ameloblastic carcinoma one observation each, respectively.

The histological grading of the tumour is an important prognostic indicator of the degree of malignancy of squamous cell carcinoma (Table 8).

Table 8. - Degree of tumour differentiation in the overall <u>cohort of patients</u>

Degree of tumour differentiation	Number of observations	%
Grade 1, highly differentiated cancer.	57	33,7
Grade 2 - moderately differentiated	90	53,2
Grade 3 - poorly differentiated	16	9,5
Grade x - differentiation not established	6	3,5
Total	169	100%

The panel of the degree of histological differentiation of tumour cells was predominantly represented by moderately differentiated tumour cells   (G2) grade

malignancy - in 90 (53.2%), and in 6 (3.5%) patients the degree of malignancy could not be determined. Discrepancy of histological data of biopsy and postoperative material was observed in 22 patients, which made 13%, and in 17 (10.0%) - the degree of tumour biopsy differentiation before surgery was G1, postoperative tumour macro preparation - G2. Conversely, in 4 (2.4%) patients, the postoperative macro preparation was found to be G2 instead of G1 preoperatively. IN 1 (0.6%) G2 - G3.

This phenomenon gives grounds to assume that in the course of treatment in certain cases malignant tumour tends to transform into a more aggressive form and, accordingly, to show resistance to methods of antitumour therapy. Sometimes the degree of differentiation cannot be revealed by morphologists at all (Gx), in our study such cases were observed in 6 (3.5%) patients. Depending on the form of tumour growth the patients were distributed as follows. Exophytic tumours occurred in 119 (76.3%) patients, endophytic tumours - in 29 (17.2%), tumours of mixed (exophytic-endophytic) growth form were detected in 21 (12.4%) patients (Table 9).

Table 9. - Distribution of patients depending on the form of tumour growth

The shape of the tumour growth	Number of observations	%
Exophytic form	119	70,4
Endophytic form	29	17,2
Mixed form	21	12,4
Total:	169	100%

Traditionally, the development of treatment tactics in patients with tumour lesions of the head and neck organs is determined collegially, with the involvement of oncological specialists (surgeons, chemotherapists, radiologists and radiation diagnosticians). A special emphasis should be placed on a differentiated approach, providing for a detailed clinical, radiological and morphological examination of patients, taking into account the localisation and spread of the tumour process, the radiation dose received and the stage of surgical treatment. The aim of the collegial approach is to reduce complications before and after the treatment process and to improve the quality of life of patients.

2.2 Research methods for assessing the general condition and quality of life of patients

Oncologists of the State Institution "RONC" of the Ministry of Health and Social Development of the Republic of Tajikistan and the staff of the Department of Oncology and Radiation Diagnostics of the Abuali Ibni Sino State Medical University of Tajikistan took part in the examination of the patients.

In both groups, patients at initial admission to the outpatient department of the RONC were examined by a head and neck tumour specialist, and in complicated cases multidisciplinary boards (Tumor board) were set up, consisting of the department curator, a professor from the Department of Oncology of the Abuali Ibni Sino State Medical University, deputy directors for medical treatment, head of the general oncology department, radiotherapists and chemotherapists to develop optimal treatment tactics.

Prior to surgery, all patients under the current protocols for diagnosis and treatment of cancer patients underwent objective clinical examination, including oroscopy, rhinoscopy, indirect laryngoscopy (fibrolaryngoscopy), comprehensive examination with determination of blood, urine, blood chemistry, coagulogram, ECG, ultrasound of the abdominal cavity and neck, review radiography of the lungs, skull bones, panoramic radiography of the jaws, CT scan of the head and neck. In cases of reversible pathology on the side of respiratory, cardiovascular and digestive systems, conservative treatment of patients was performed.

All patients were examined in accordance with the accepted algorithm for this category of patients, including blood tests (general and biochemical), urine, consultation with a general practitioner, cardiologist, anaesthesiologist and other specialists if indicated. Additional instrumental methods of examination, as well as methods of radiation diagnostics were performed as indicated.

Within the framework of the approved national standards of treatment of MND, patients of both groups received treatment after discussion and approval of the developed tactics at the medical conference, where specialists of all oncology profiles participated. The scope of treatment of patients included: Preoperative radiotherapy (RT) with subsequent operation in total 63 (37,3%) patients - 33 patients of the main group and 30 patients of the control group. Chemoradiotherapy (CRT) with subsequent surgery was given to 37 (21.9%) patients, of which 25 patients from the main group and 12 from the control group. Neoadjuvant chemotherapy (NCT) followed by surgery was given to 17 (10.0%) patients, of whom 13 were in the main group and 4 in the control group.

Surgery followed by radiotherapy (RT) at 3-4 weeks after surgery was performed in 31 (18.3%) patients, of whom 21 were from the main group and 10 from the control group. Surgery followed by chemotherapy at 3 weeks postoperatively was performed in 11 (6.0%) patients, of whom 9 were from the main group and 2 from the control group. Also, 10 (5.9%)

patients, 7 from the main group and 3 from the control group, underwent only surgical intervention (Table 10).

Table 10. - Tactics of treatment of patients

Treatment methods	Main group, abs. number, (%)		Control group, abs. number, (%)		Total abs. number, (%)	P
LT + Operation	33		30		63 (37,3%)	0,006
hlt + Operation	25	71 (65,7%)	12	46 (75,4%)	37 (22,0%)	0,600
XT + Surgery	13		4		17 (10,0%)	0,384
Total	117 (69,2%), p = 0,191					
Surgery + LT	21	30 (27,8%)	10	12 (19,7%)	31 (18,3%)	0,972
Surgery + XT	9		2		11 (6,5%)	0,340
Total	42 (24,9%),		p = 0,242			
Operation Total	7	6,5%	3	4,9%	10 (5,9%)	0,680
	10 (5,9%), p = 0,941					

Note: p - statistical significance of the difference between the indicators of the main and control groups (by Pearson's $\%^2$ criterion).

The majority of patients n=117 (69.2%) underwent surgical intervention at the second stage - after neoadjuvant radiation, chemotherapy and chemoradiotherapy. The proportion of this category was 71 (65.7%) in the main group and 46 (75.4%) in the control group.

Surgical intervention preceded adjuvant radiotherapy and chemotherapy in 42 patients (24.9%), of whom 30 (27.8%) were in the main group and 12 (19.7%) in the control group. Only 10 (5.9%) patients underwent surgical intervention alone.

It is recommended to assess the general condition of cancer patients using the Karnofsky Index (0-100%) or the ECOG-Performance Status Scale (0-4 points). In this case, complaints, presence or absence of symptoms, physical activity of the patient, need for special medical care are assessed.

To characterise simple quality of life (QOL) parameters, we evaluated the initial condition of patients before and after surgical intervention. For this purpose, the general condition of patients before and after the surgical stage of treatment was determined using the Karnovsky scale (0-100 points) (Table 11).

Table 11. - Karnofsky index

Scores	Characterisation
Normal physical activity, the patient does not need special care	
100%	Condition is normal, no complaints or symptoms of illness
90%	Normal activity is preserved, but minor symptoms of the disease are present
80%	Normal activity is possible with extra effort, with moderately severe symptoms of the disease
Restriction of normal activity while maintaining the patient's complete independence	
70%	The patient maintains self-care but is unable to perform normal activities or work
60%	The patient sometimes needs help, but is mostly self-cared for
50%	The patient often requires assistance and medical care
The patient is unable to care for himself/herself and requires nursing care or hospitalisation	
40%	The patient spends most of the time in bed, special care and assistance is required
30%	The patient is bedridden and hospitalisation is indicated, although a terminal condition is not necessary
20%	Severe manifestations of the disease, hospitalisation is necessary and supportive therapy
10%	Dying patient, rapid progression of the disease
0%	Death

Clinical trials of different treatments for malignant neoplasms require the use of standardised criteria to measure how the disease affects the patient's daily activities. Consequently, we also applied the ECOG scale (0-4 points) to investigate the outcome of patients in both groups. The ECOG scale is one of the tools to describe the patient's level of functional status in terms of self-care ability, daily activities and physical activity (walking, working, etc.). This scale was developed by the Eastern Cooperative Oncology Group (ECOG), which is now part of the ECOG- ACRIN Cancer Research Group. Researchers around the world consider ECOG status when planning studies to investigate a new treatment. This scale allows the results of studies to be reproduced (Table 12).

Table 12. - Evaluation of the general condition of the patient according to the ECOG scale

Scores	Characterisation
0	The patient is fully active, able to do everything as before the disease (90-100% on the Karnofsky scale)
1	The patient is unable to do heavy work but can do light or sedentary work (e.g., light housework or clerical work, 7080% on the Karnofsky scale)
2	The patient is treated as an outpatient, is capable of
	Self-care, but cannot perform work. Spends more than 50 per cent of waking time active - in an upright position (5060 per cent on the Karnofsky scale)
3	The patient is capable of only limited self-care, spends more than 50% of waking time in a chair or bed (30-40% on the Karnofsky scale)
4	Disabled, totally incapable of self-care, confined to a chair or bed (10-20% on the Karnofsky scale)

The state of quality of life in the pre- and postoperative periods was also assessed using the EORTC-QLQ-30 questionnaires and a special module designed for head and neck tumours EORTC QLQ H&N35, version 3.0. In our study, the EORTC-QLQ H&N35 scale was applied for the first time in the Republic. The results of the study emphasise the direct change in the parameters of patients' quality of life before and after the surgical stage of head and neck cancer treatment, which are expressed by the patients themselves in quantitative form.

The European Organisation for Research and Treatment of Cancer Quality of Life Questionnaire (EORTC-QLQ-C30) is designed to assess quality of life parameters in patients with advanced cancer. A distinctive feature of this questionnaire is that it is available in 9 different languages (Belgium, Denmark, France, Germany, the Netherlands, England, Australia, Canada and Japan). This questionnaire includes 30 questions consisting of 9 scales. After receiving the answers to the questions, this questionnaire is subjected to mathematical processing according to the formula:

$$1 - (RS - 1) / range \ x \ 100,$$

where RS (Raw Score) is the sum of scores in relation to the number of questions of the given scale, range is the difference between the maximum and minimum values of the answer to the question. Scale values ranged from 0 to 100.

Symptom scales are scored using the following formula:

$$(RS - 1) / range \ x \ 100,$$

Analysis of the results suggests that high scores indicate a high level of EF for the functional scales and symptom severity for the symptom scales.

EORTC has developed a new EORTC-QLQ-H&N35 version 3.0 questionnaire to assess quality of life in patients with head and neck cancer. This questionnaire is intended for use in international cancer clinical trials as a standardised tool for assessing quality of life in patients with HNC. The QLQ-H&N35 questionnaire includes 35 items and consists of 18 scales, of which 7 scales with multiple items: pain, swallowing, sensory, and speech impairment, eating difficulties , social functioning, sex drive, and 11 scales with 1 item: dental problems, limitation of mouth opening, dry mouth, salivary viscosity, coughing, feeling generally sore, pain management, taking supplements, using a nasogastric tube, weight loss and gain.

The scores for each scale range from 0 to 100, where for the functional subscale higher scores indicate better conditions, and for the symptom scale higher scores indicate, on the contrary, more severe symptoms. This questionnaire has been translated and adapted by us into the state Tajik language, formalised as an act of implementation in the treatment process of oncological institutions.

Thus, methods and approaches to assessing the QoL of oncological patients have a wide range of possibilities, carrying different volumes of interpretation. Many authors note that the effectiveness of cancer treatment is measured not only by survival and life expectancy, but also by equally important quality of life parameters. For this reason, rehabilitation programmes are often developed on the basis of QOL indicators. The follow-up period of the patients ranged from 1.4 to 60 months. Survival data were traced from attendance records at the outpatient department of the RONC, which was supplemented in retrospective patients by telephone interview of the patients' family members.

Statistical analysis of the results was performed using the application programme "Statistica 10.0" (Stat Soft Inc., USA). Absolute values were presented as median and lower with upper quartile (Me [25q; 75q]), and relative values were presented as fractions (%). Comparison of absolute values for dependent samples was performed using the Wilcoxon T-criterion, for independent samples - using the Mann-Whitney U-criterion. Comparison of relative values for dependent samples was carried out using the $\%^2$ McNemar criterion, and for independent samples - using Pearson's $\%^2$. The null

hypothesis was rejected at p <0.05. Evaluation of terminal actions (survival-mortality,
the onset of complications) was analysed using the Kaplan-Meier graphical method. Comparisons were made using the Cox criterion.

CHAPTER 3

METHODS OF RECONSTRUCTION OF HEAD AND NECK DEFECTS AFTER TUMOUR REMOVAL

3.1 Characterisation of defects forming on the head and neck after cancer surgery

When developing the treatment plan, the method of reconstruction must be planned at the same time. It is fundamentally important to determine the volume of reconstruction simultaneously with the surgical intervention. When the postoperative defect is large, it is advisable to use arterialised flaps [115].

Indications and contraindications for performing one-stage reconstructive-reconstructive surgery.

head and neck cancer surgeries are determined on the basis of the following criteria: a group of factors relating to the malignancy: Localisation, tumour size (according to the symbol T), singularity or multiplicity of the primary tumour, stage of the malignant tumour and its histological structure, relationship with underlying structures, cranial bones, depth of invasion, growth form, status of regional lymph nodes (criterion N), previous preoperative chemo-radiation therapy, estimated volume of tissues to be removed during surgery and patient-related factors - age, gender, general somatic status of patients, i.e. the presence or absence of comorbidities, lifestyle, oral hygiene, occupation, profession.i.e. presence or absence of comorbidities, lifestyle, oral hygiene, occupation, awareness of the seriousness of the disease, tolerance, patient compliance with the operating surgeon's instructions, socio-economic factors and time constraints. Hence, there is a need to scrutinise these factors prior to surgical intervention.

An important point is the study of the characteristics of the resulting defects, such as: the size of the defect, its localisation, the type of tissue at the bottom of the defect formed. In the case of through defects, a clear description of the nature of the epithelial surfaces limiting the defect is necessary. It is important to emphasise that a clinico-anatomically sound and at the same time accessible working classification of the defects formed is necessary for optimal flap selection.

There are many classifications, the underlying factors of which are: division of the face into anatomical quadrants, localisation of the defect, size of the defect, organ or group of organs to be removed [68]. These classifications are not very practical and difficult to apply in practice. One of the problems in planning defect reconstruction is the surgeon's subjective judgement in determining the volume of resection and the optimality of the selected flap, which can lead to postoperative complications and poor results (functional and cosmetic).

Reconstruction of defects of head and neck organs involves manipulations in two epithelial coverings that differ in structure and function - skin and oral mucous membranes. Many studies have proved that skin in the form of a free full-layer flap or as a component of an arterialised flap is used to close defects of both skin and mucous membranes, which over time acquires the property of local tissues.

Consequently, this further supports the need to use a simplified and unified clinical classification of defects.

We adhere to the classification proposed by Khabibulaev Sh.Z. (2011), which clinically has been tested in our patients. The following types of postoperative defects requiring one-stage reconstruction are formed as a result of combined and extended combined operations for head and neck cancer:

I category of defects - Non-cavitary defects of skin, muscle and bone tissues that do not communicate with cavities. These defects are usually formed after excision of parotid-cervical skin cancer, parotid salivary gland cancer with skin involvement, cheek cancer, skin cancer of the scalp, neck, etc. (Figure 20).

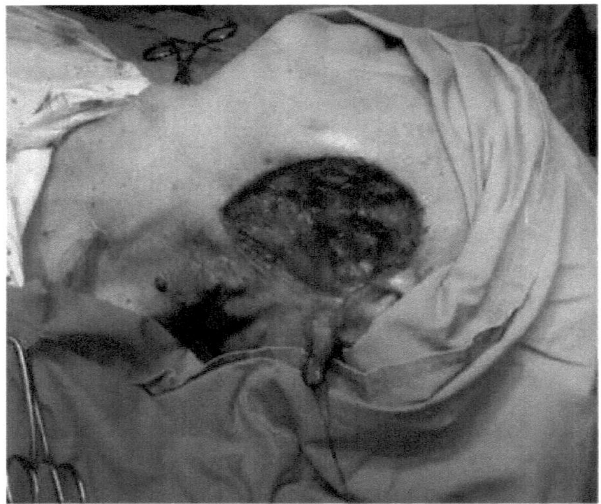

Figure 20. - Patient X., 75 years old. Medical history #4169. Diagnosis: Cancer of the left parotid-cervical region T4N0M0. Defect of the parotid-mandibular region. The block of tissues to be removed includes: skin, subcutaneous fat layer, parotid salivary gland, partially auricle, part of the masseter muscle

Category II defects - non-contiguous defects of mucous membranes, muscles and bones with preserved skin. These include defects after excision of cancer of the oral cavity, lip mucosa, and nasal cavities (Figure 21).

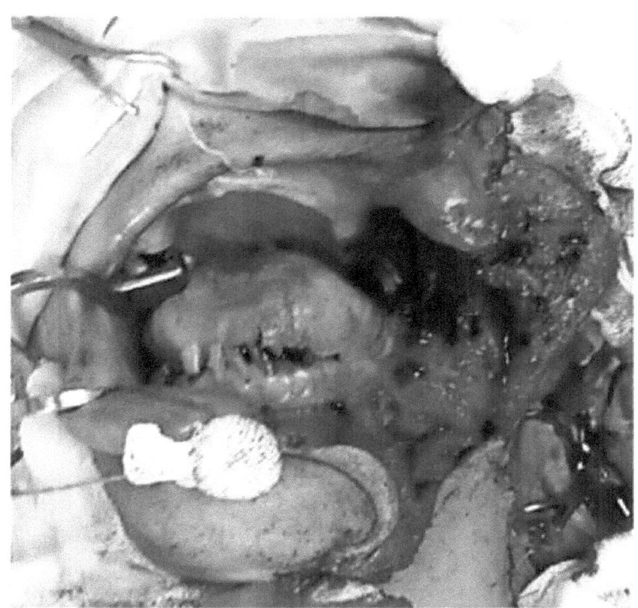

Figure 21. - Patient K., 56 years old. Case history #2617. Defect of the mucosa and soft tissues of the retromolar region of the left cheek in the absence of skin lesions, operated for recurrent cancer of the left cheek mucosa, spreading to the alveolar process of the upper cheek.

jaws

III category of defects - Through defects of mucous membranes, muscle and bone defects communicating with the skin surface over a large length. These include penetrating defects after excision of cancer of the oral cavity, lower and upper lips, nasal cavity and maxillary sinus, which sprout and infiltrate the skin (Figure 22).

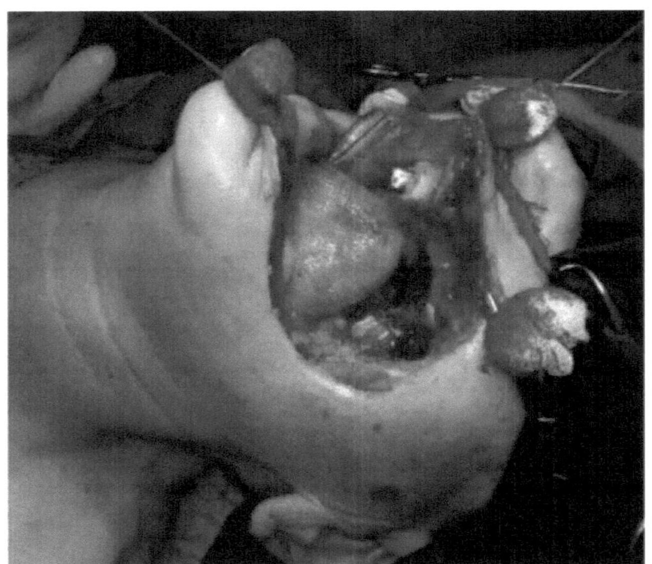

Figure 22. - Patient M., 60 years old, case history №1997. Extensive penetrating defect of the mucosa, soft tissues and skin of the left cheek area, operated for left cheek mucosal cancer T4N0M0, stage IV

The IV category of defects is through defects of the larynx and pharynx, so-called laryngostomas and pharyngostomas. These include laryngostomas and pharyngostomas formed for laryngeal and thyroid cancer (Figure 23).

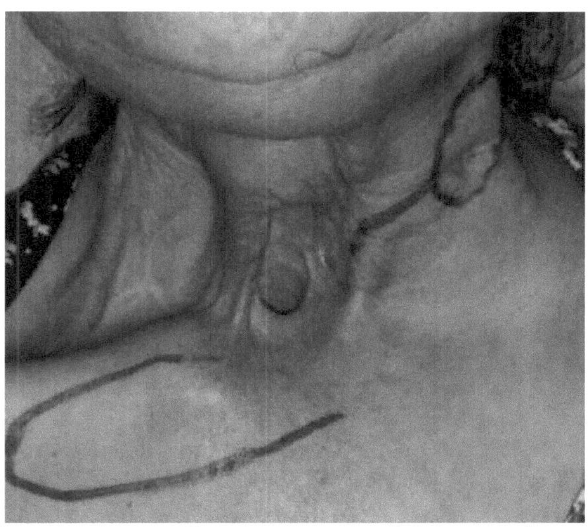

Figure 23. - Patient S., 65 years old, case history #3580. Through tracheal defect in a patient 6 months after thyroidectomy for thyroid cancer with sprouting into the trachea. A section of the anterior wall of the trachea is missing along the four cartilaginous semicondyles

V category of defects - Through defects of the scalp skin communicating with the cranial cavity, when the tumour affects the scalp skin with penetration and destruction of the cranial bones up to the dura mater.

The first category of defects included 36 (21.3%) patients with primary and recurrent skin cancer of different localisations of the head and neck, parotid salivary gland, as well as 1 patient with locally spread cancer of the parotid salivary gland sprouting adjacent skin and muscles. Of these, 24 (66.7%) patients belonged to the main group and 12 (33.4%) patients belonged to the control group. Among them, 25 were males and 11 were females. Here we are talking about simple skin defects when the tissues to be excised include skin, subcutaneous fat fibres up to the intrinsic fascia of the muscle, and sometimes the periosteum. Often the bottom of deeper defects formed are any non-epithelial tissues and anatomical formations of the head and neck (skin wound edges, subcutaneous fatty layer, muscles, skull bones, various glandular elements of the skin and some anatomical formations (external ear canal, large vessels and nerves of the head and neck) (Figure 20).

Table 15. - Distribution of category I defects <u>depending on tumour stage</u>

TNM / localisation of the defect	T2N0M0	T2N1M0	T3N0M0	T3N1M0	T3N2M0	T4N0M0	T4N1M0	T4N2M0	Total
Scalp	1	-	2	-	-	3	3	-	9
Cheekbone region	2	-	1	2	-	1	-	-	6
Auricular skin	-	-	-	-	-	5	1	1	7
Nasal skin	-	-	3	-	-	2	-	-	5
Periradicular region	-	-	-	-	-	4	-	-	4
The skin of the cheek	-	-	1	-	-	1	-	-	2
The skin of the forehead	-	-	1	-	-	-	-	-	1
Eyelid skin	-	-	-	-	-	1	-	-	1
Neck skin	-	-	-	-	-	1	-	-	1
Total:	3	-	8	2	-	18	4	1	36

The data in Table 15 show that the highest incidence of category 1 defects occurred after surgery for scalp and malar skin cancer in 15 (41.6%) cases, auricle and skin of various subunits of the nose in 7 and 5 cases, respectively (19.4% and 13.8%).

In 3 (8.3%) patients, the tumour stage corresponded to the T2 symbol, and in 23 (91%) patients - locally T3 - 10 (27.7%) and T4 - 23 (63.8%). Of these, metastases in regional lymph nodes were diagnosed in 7 (19.4%) observations at the initial treatment of patients. These were 2 patients diagnosed with skin cancer of the right zygomatic area and 2 patients with skin cancer of the auricle, who underwent combined and complex treatment with the final stage of extended surgery.

The second category of defects was established in 116

(68.6%) patients with cancer of the lip and oral cavity, of which 70 (60.8%) patients belonged to the main group and 46 (39.2%) patients in the control group, in which 101 (87.8%) cases had locally advanced tumour process of stage III-IV (Table 16).

Table 16. - Localisation of category II defects by primary tumour stage in patients of the main/ and control groups

TNM / defect localisation	T2N0M0	T2N1M0	T3N0M0	T3N1M0	T3N2M0	T4N0M0	T4N1M0	T4N2M0	Total	
Alv. process of the mandible	1/0	-	2/1	1/1	-	7/2	7/4	2/3	20/11	31
Language	1/5	-	1/4	1/3	1/1	1/0	0/1	2/2	7/16	23
Cheek	2/1	-	3/1	5/0	1/0	4/0	4/0	-	19/2	21
Lips	4/0	1/0	3/0	2/0	-	2/0	1/1	-	13/1	14
The floor of the mouth	-	-	1/0	2/0	0/1	1/1	3/0	2/0	9/2	11
Upper jaw	-	-	0/2	-	-	0/8	-	-	0/10	10
The alveolar process of the maxilla.	-	-	-	-	-	1/4	1/0	-	2/4	6
Total	14	1	18	15	4	31	22	11	70/46	116

There were 68 males (58.6%) and 48 females (41.4%) with a ratio of 1:1.4. As a result of combined and extended combined surgeries, these patients had complex defects of the oral mucosa, underlying muscles and subcutaneous tissue, including the mucosa, underlying muscles to the subcutaneous fat layer, and sometimes to the skin. The main feature of this group of defects is the need to close only one epithelial surface in the absence of skin lesions.

The most difficult category of defects **is the third group** in terms of preoperative preparation, determination of tactics and time of reconstruction. The localisation of category III defects and the stage of the tumour process are shown in Table 17.

Table 17. - Localisation of category III defects by primary tumour stage in patients of the main/ and control groups

˄˄˄˄˄˄˄˄˄˄.TNM stage	T3N1	T3N2	T4N0	T4N1	T4N2	Total

Localisation Defect						
Alveolar process of the mandible	-	-	-	3/0	2/0	5/0
Upper jaw	-	1/0	0/3	-	-	1/3
Cheek mucosa	2/0	-	1/0	-	1	4/0
The red border of the lower lip	-	-	1/0	-	-	1/0
Total	2	1	5	3	3	11/3 (14)

Defects of the third category were formed in 14 (8.3%) patients with locally advanced cancer of the maxilla and nasal cavities, oral cavity organs, and lip. Of them 11 (78,5%) patients from the main group underwent flap plasty and 3 (21,5%) patients from the control group underwent local tissue plasty of the defect. Of the 14 patients, 9 (64.3%) already had regional metastases in lymph nodes at the time of admission for treatment.

All patients underwent combined and extended combined operations after tumour removal, which resulted in extensive penetrating defects of soft tissues and bones, for the closure of which more than one flap on a pedicle was required in 4 (40%) cases: the first - to form the inner lining of the oral cavity, the second - to restore the integrity of the skin. In three cases with the diagnosis of locally advanced cancer of the mucosa of the mandibular alveolar process, a musculoskeletal BGM flap was used in combination with a skin-fat cervical flap - 1 case, with a deltopectoral flap - 1 case, and a musculoskeletal BGM flap with a fragment of the V-rib with a musculoskeletal subclavian and chin flap. In 1 case, the extensive defect included a mental fragment of the mandibular bone, which is the most difficult for reconstruction, where in addition to the BGM, a sublingual flap with a subchondral musculocutaneous flap was used.

Thus, cancer was most often localised in the alveolar process of the mandible - in 5 cases. With equal frequency - 4 cases each in the maxilla and cheek mucosa. Only in 1 patient the tumour was located on the red border of the lower lip, growing through its entire thickness and the skin of the chin.

The group of patients **with IV category of defects** in our study was represented by a relatively smaller number - 3 (1.8%) patients. Of them, 2 (66.6%) patients had verified laryngeal cancer, who underwent combined and complex treatment - anterolateral resection of the larynx with the formation of a planned laryngostomy, and the plastic stage was performed after a six-month follow-up to exclude recurrence. As a plastic material we used a skin-muscular flap of platysma. One patient (33.4%) had thyroid cancer with sprouting into the trachea, who underwent a combined operation for removal of the primary tumour with formation of a permanent tracheostomy. The restorative stage of chondroplasty according to the Koenig method was performed 6 months later. The essence of this method is the use of a cartilage fragment to form a tracheal framework. As the latter we used a fragment of tissue from the thyroid cartilage. Reconstruction of this kind of defects is the only example of delayed plasty, also belonging to combined methods, including the formation of two epithelial surfaces: the inner covering playing the role of the mucous membrane (larynx or trachea), the outer one forming a defect of the proper skin of the anterior surface of the neck (Figure 24).

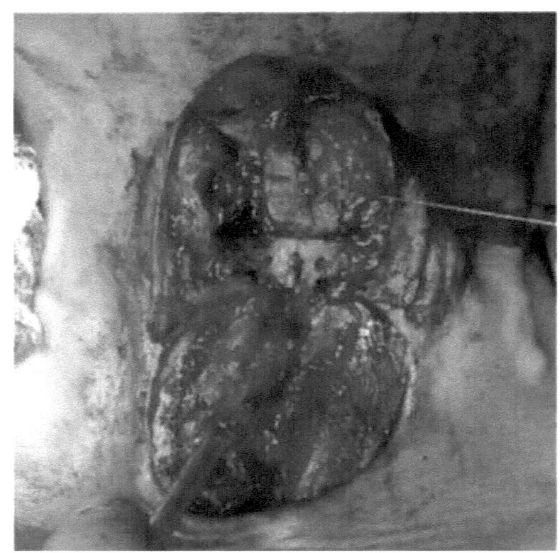

Figure 24. - Patient S., 65 years old, medical history #3580. Plasty of a through tracheal defect in a patient 6 months after thyroidectomy with tracheal resection for locally advanced thyroid cancer with tracheal growth into the trachea

As it has been already mentioned 48 (44,4%) patients of the main group and 21 (34,4%) patients of the control group had cancer metastases in regional lymph nodes. In these cases lymphodissection was performed in the following volumes: Unilateral fascial-futlar excision of the neck fibre (n = 39) was performed in 32 patients of the main group and 7 patients of the control group. Kreil's operation from one side (n = 24) was performed in 17 patients of the main group and 7 patients of the control group. Of them one patient from the main group along with the Kreil's operation on the right side underwent FFICC on the opposite side. The upper variant of unilateral FFIKSH (n = 13) was performed in 7 patients of the main group and 6 patients of the control group. Bilateral FVFCS (n = 5) was performed in 3 patients of the main group and 1 patient of the control group. The upper variant of bilateral FFIKSH (n = 3) was performed in 2 patients of the main group and 1 patient of the control group. Selective lymphodissection (n = 3) was performed in 2 patients of the main group and 1 patient from the control group.

Two types of reconstructive and reconstructive surgeries are mainly used to repair complex defects after tumour removal for locally advanced head and neck cancer:

1. Formation of vascularised flaps with preservation of the blood supply source close to the defect.

2. Free transplantation of tissue complexes with immediate revascularisation by microvascular anastomosis.

The latter is more complex and expensive. This type of plastic surgery is widely used in practice, especially optimal for bone grafting of mandibular defects, which uses tissue complexes with the inclusion of fibula, iliac crest, outer edge of the scapula, radius, rib fragment. This method of defect plasty in our country is performed mainly in the specialised republican centre of reconstructive and plastic surgery. To introduce this technique into oncological practice in the future, close scientific and practical cooperation of interested structures is necessary.

3.2 Topographic and anatomical description of the pedicled flaps used for plasty

postoperative defects

To replace the formed postoperative defects, we used complex skin-fat, skin-fascial, skin-muscular and skin-muscular-bone vascularised flaps with axial blood flow. In these flaps, the main functional load falls on the skin "island" left on the distal fragment of the skin-fat and skin-muscular flap, which reliably protects all the underlying structures and well resists various factors of the external and internal environment. In the proximal section, the flap pedicle plays the role of a base through which the skin islet and the flap as a whole are nourished.

The main aims of head and neck defect reconstruction are to restore as close to normal in appearance and function as possible, minimising any additional incisions and trauma.

The correct choice of the type of plastic material to replace defects of the head and neck depends on many factors: the history of the disease and previously used methods of treatment, the histological structure of the tumour, the stage of the tumour process, the shape, localisation and extensiveness of the defect, the viability of the donor bed, and the prognosis of the disease. It is also necessary to take into account the experience and preference of the surgeon, the patient's motivation, i.e. the patient's desire for a good result, the patient's general condition, the presence or absence of vascular pathology. All these factors should be clarified before surgery, as the presence of one or a combination of these factors is decisive in choosing the optimal flap to obtain the best oncological and aesthetic results.

The use of vascularised flaps has its advantages and disadvantages: Firstly, plasty with a vascularised flap is performed simultaneously with the removal of the malignant tumour, which significantly reduces the treatment time. Secondly, it expands the indications of surgical intervention, as these flaps can be used to close almost all types of defects, which creates the possibility of radical excision of the affected tissues. Thirdly, the use of vascularised flap significantly improves blood circulation in the surrounding tissues, which is extremely important for faster healing, fighting infection, etc. Fourthly, the use of a vascularised flap does not require prolonged immobilisation. Another equally important factor is the similarity, and sometimes similarity of the donor graft to the surrounding defect tissues - these are such properties as the skin colour of the flap, its pigmentation degree, dermographism, presence (and sometimes absence) of hair cover, severity of subcutaneous tissue, saturation of sebaceous and sweat glands, etc.

The above factors should be mainly taken into account in the plasty of extensive defects of the face and neck, which are also of aesthetic importance. In this way, better functional and cosmetic results can be achieved, which is extremely important for improving the quality of life of patients. To cover large vessels and nerve trunks of the neck region from potential drying, infection, and arterial bleeding after cervical fibre excision surgeries, the muscular part of the flap can be used, which serves as a base.

Not all oncosurgeons are in favour of reconstruction, and they perform operations using displaced skin flaps taken in close proximity to the edges of the defect. This approach often creates a lot of inconvenience and requires additional incisions in the open areas of the head and neck, thereby breaking the symmetry of the latter with tight skin fragments and the appearance of rough postoperative scars. In addition, it should be taken into account the fact that adjacent to the tumour and the defect formed after its removal tissues are often included in the field of radiation in patients who received the maximum permissible dose of radiation therapy. In these tissues normal blood supply is often disturbed, metabolic and regenerative-restorative processes are reduced, therefore, it prevents complete healing of the flap. We consider it most appropriate and give preference to flaps that are localised in "intact" areas that have not been exposed to radiation.

The use of vascularised flaps on a pedicle with an axial type of blood circulation is the simplest method to achieve high functional and aesthetic results. The success of flap plasty of postoperative defects depends entirely on the state of their blood circulation. The main characteristic of vascularised flaps is considered to be the peculiarities of blood supply of the graft tissues. Numerous clinical researches proved that if the length and width ratios of 1:1 - 1:1,5 are observed, the flaps can be displaced without the danger of necrosis, and wider cutting off of the flaps leads to a pronounced hypoxia of the end sections. Therefore, the rule of length and width compliance is an important point in reconstructive surgery.

Currently, there are descriptions in the literature of many different flaps that can be used for reconstructive surgery. These flaps are classified according to different principles, but basically the whole arsenal of flaps is divided into two main groups:

1. arterialised flaps on a feeding pedicle.

2. Free on a vascular pedicle.

Depending on the tissue structures represented, these flaps can be skin-fat, skin-fascial, skin-muscle, and skin-muscle-bone. Their distinction from each other is related to the provision of nutrition to the flaps. The use of free flaps is possible if precision technology and trained personnel are available.

Also the varieties of free flaps include the flap of the greater omentum, fragments of the small intestine and cecum with the adjacent sector of the mesentery, which are widely used in the reconstruction of the circular oncological defect of the pharynx. According to the distance of the donor site from the recipient site, they are divided into local, regional and distant flaps. According to the structure and type of tissue from which the flap is composed, skin, skin-fascial, skin-fat, skin-fat, skin-muscle, skin-muscle-bone, pure muscle and bone flaps are distinguished.

The most common classification of flaps is based on the principles of structure and the nature of their blood supply.

According to the principle according to which vessels penetrate into the flap at its base, they are divided into flaps with axial (axial) and random (chaotic) type of blood supply. Axial flaps are supplied with blood mainly by the eponymous cutaneous or saphenous arteries and veins, which penetrate the thickness of the flap throughout its entire length. This type of blood supply contributes to the nourishment of a relatively large area of tissues, where compliance with the technique of flap harvesting with preservation of axial vessels, the need to take into account the ratio of length and width as a limiting factor is not mandatory (Figure 25).

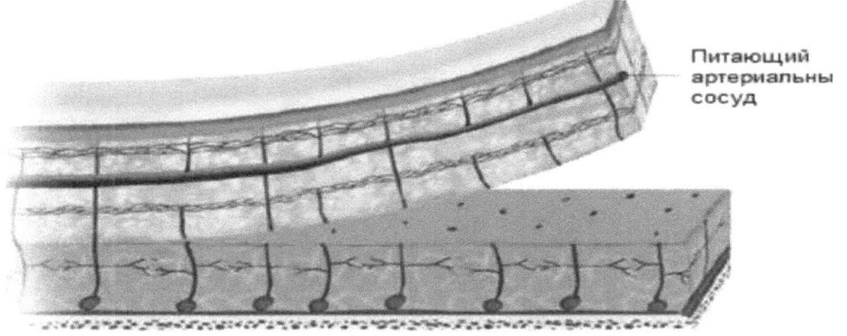

Figure 25. - Schematic drawing of the flap structure with axial type of blood supply

The nutrition of disordered flaps is based on a plexus of subcutaneous vessels that are supplied by perforating vessels that penetrate the flap at its base. To ensure survival in the facial region, these flaps must be cut with a length-to-width ratio not exceeding 3:1. However, the survival of the flap depends not only on its length but also on perfusion pressure and intravascular resistance   , which play an important role (Fig. 26).

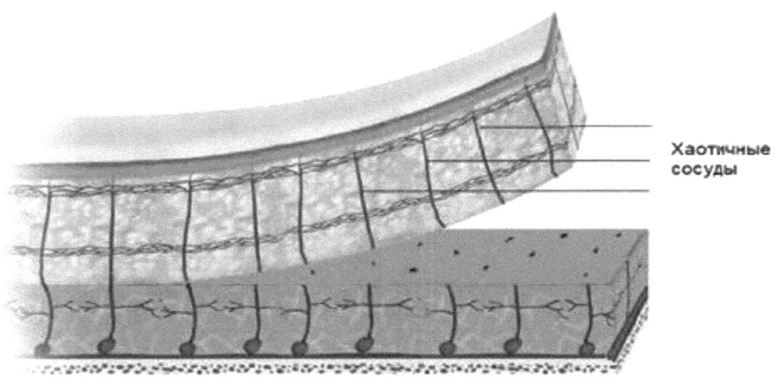

Figure 26. - Schematic drawing of the flap structure with disordered type of blood supply

Our study presents the results of using autologous flaps on the feeding pedicle and free split skin grafts. The term "feeding pedicle" refers to the base of the graft, which has blood vessels, through which the functionally significant distal end of the flap - the skin islet - is trophised. In some cases the flap pedicle is formed only as a base, and it is excised after the working distal part of the flap is fully engrafted and the autonomous blood supply develops in it. However, in all of the above cases, the main load is borne by the skin islet of the flap, which fulfils a protective role in the reconstruction of defects.

3.3 Selection of the optimal method of plasty depending on the anatomo-topographical characteristics of the flaps, localisation and category of defects

Flap engraftment and integration depends on a number of factors, in particular, on the anatomo-topographical structure and the nature of the blood supply, which allows the flap to be raised to the length of the axial vessel. Dermatofat flaps, which include only skin and subcutaneous fatty tissue, are the thinnest, due to this fact, the vessels, located superficially, provide blood supply to a small area of skin. However, due to their vulnerability, these flaps are limitedly used to replace defects of the oral cavity and oropharynx mucosa.

When taking skin-fat flaps, it is preferable to model the flap, taking into account the specific location of superficial capillary vessels that are unevenly distributed in the subcutaneous tissue, which often rupture if the flap is handled carelessly. Consequently, skin-fat flaps need to be lifted together with the underlying superficial fascia, resulting in skin-fascial flaps. In contrast to the skin and fat flaps, the cutaneous fascial flaps are characterised by better blood supply and grafting. The superficial fascia in this case plays the role of a barrier to the back surface of the flap, facilitates the preparation of the flap and ensures the preservation of the vascular network throughout its entire length. Depending on which fascia is included in the flap component, superficial and deep cutaneous fascial flaps are distinguished.

Safavi A. et al. (2015) an experimental study was conducted to investigate the vascular anatomy of different musculoskeletal, dermal-fascial and mucosal flaps on human cadavers.

They used blue and red colloidal substance on silicone-rubber base to outline the vascular network, after which the flaps were dissected. When the results were evaluated, they found that colloid accumulation in the flaps listed was up to 90%, and this figure was dramatically reduced to 20% when the fascia was dissected. The authors concluded that knowledge of the surgical anatomy of the head and neck is crucial, and preserving the fascial layers of the flaps can reduce the incidence of specific complications by up to 70%. Therefore, only skin-fascial or so-called "complex flaps" are preferable for plasty of extensive defects of the head and neck.

The variety and frequency of grafts used in our study are summarised in Table 18.

Table 18. – Variety and frequency of grafts used

№	Types of flaps	Number of	Total

		flaps	
Musculoskeletal flaps comprising:			
1	Large pectoral muscle (LMP).	37	**65 (49,2%)**
2	Sternoclavicular-papillary (SCP).	12	
3	Sternal hyoid (SG).	12	
4	Platysma (PL)	3	
5	Trapezoidal (TP)	1	
Percutaneous fascial and cutaneous fat flaps			
1	Nasolabial (NG)	32	**56 (42,4%)**
2	Cervical (NF)	7	
3	Frontal	5	
4	Submental	4	
5	Temporal	3	
6	Deltopectoral	2	
7	Cutaneous fascial from the behind-the-ear region	2	
8	Temennoi	1	
Other flaps			
1	Free split skin flap	8	**11 (8,2%)**
2	Cheek mucosal flap	3	
	Total		**132 (100%)**

The data presented in table 18 reflect the need   for reconstruction and rehabilitation.

surgeries using one or another type of plastic material in the treatment of head and neck cancer. A total of 132 different flaps were used in our study to reconstruct head and neck defects after cancer surgery in 108 patients. Of these, skin-muscle grafts were used in 65 (49.2%) cases, and skin-fat and skin-fascial flaps were used in 56 (42.4%). The data on the use of 8 free split skin autografts and 3 cheek mucosa flaps, which accounted for 8.2%, were also included in a separate group. Combined plasty was performed in 20 patients, respectively, the number of flaps used does not coincide with the number of operated patients.

Thus, the most frequently used flaps in our study were musculocutaneous flaps. This is not a coincidence, as complex defects need to be replaced with massive muscle grafts, which are characterised by musculocutaneous flaps. Of these, flaps with the inclusion of the large pectoral muscle (LPM) accounted for 56.9%, and of the total plastic material used in reconstructive surgeries - 27.8%, which emphasises the universality of this type of flap in reconstructive oncosurgery of the head and neck, especially in oropharyngeal cancer.

The second and third most frequently used musculoskeletal flaps for defect reconstruction were skin-muscle grafts with the inclusion of the sternoclavicular-papillary and sterno hyoid muscles - in 9.9% and 9.1% of cases, respectively. Their frequent use was favoured by such characteristics as relative simplicity of the flap cutting technique and close proximity to the defect zone. Other types of musculoskeletal flaps: neck saphenous muscle flap, trapezius flap were used relatively less frequently. Among the cutaneous fascial and cutaneous-fat flaps most frequently used in our work we can list the nasolabial flap - 32 (flaps). Taking into account the localisation, this flap was used for reconstruction of facial, lower lip and oral cavity skin defects. Almost with the same frequency the plasty was performed using the cervical, frontal and submental dermofascial flaps (7; 5; and 4 cases). Temporal, deltopectoral and behind-the-ear skin-fascial flaps were used with the lowest frequency (3; 2 and 2 cases, respectively), and in one patient the scalp skin defect was restored with a parietal flap.

In order to study and compare the results of plasty, we divided all the defects formed in patients after tumour excision into 3 large groups, which are shown in Table 19.

Table 19. - Distribution of patients by defect localisation

Localisation of the defect	Main group	Control group	Total
Oral cavity, cavities nose	66 (61,1%)	45 (73,8%)	111 (65,6%)
	$P =$	0.096	
Face	32 (29,6%)	11 (18,0%)	43 (38,5%)
	$P =$	0.097	
Cranial vault and neck	10 (9,3%)	5 (8,2%)	15 (8,9%)
	$P =$	0.962	
Total	108 (100%)	61 (100%)	169 (100%)

Note: p - statistical significance of the difference between the indicators of the main and control groups (by Pearson's $\%^2$ criterion).

As can be seen from Table 20, the main share of defects in both the main and control groups was formed in the organs of the oral cavity and nose - 61.1% and 73.8%, respectively. This is explained by the fact that in the head and neck region in the structure of morbidity cancer of the oral cavity occupies the leading place. Somewhat less frequently the defects are localised in the facial region, the frequency of which is 29.6% in the main group and 18.0% in the control group. The smallest number of observed patients, defects are found on the skin of the cranial vault and neck area - 9.3% in the main group and 8.2% in the control group of cases. We have developed an algorithm for reconstruction of head and neck defects depending on the anatomo-topogaphic characteristics of the flaps, localisation and category of defect complexity (Fig. 27).

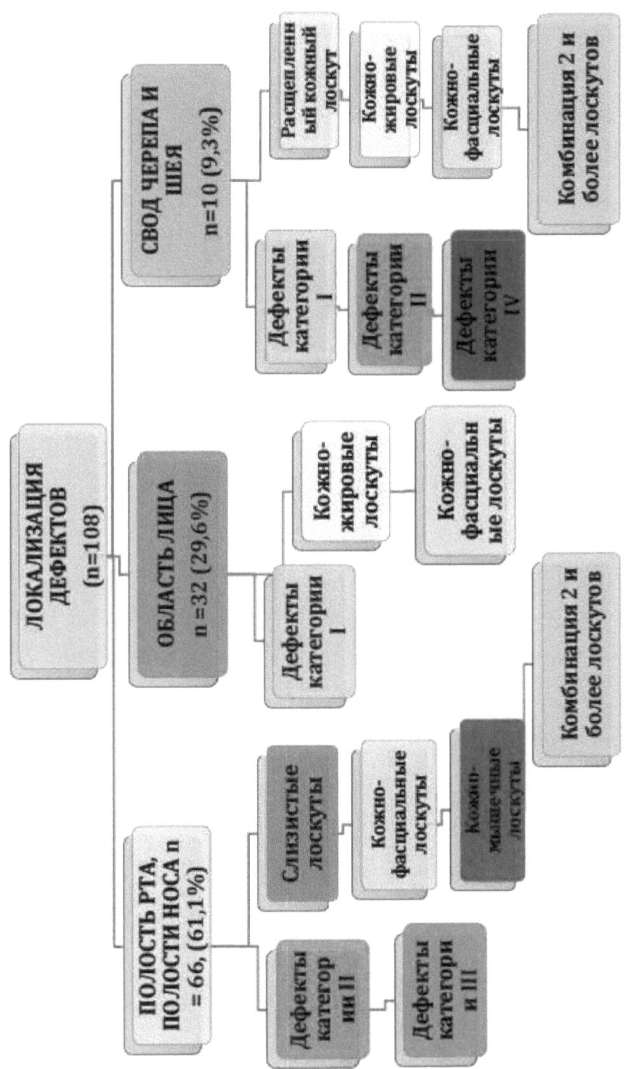

Figure 27. - Algorithm of reconstruction of postoperative defects

3.4 Comparative characterisation of pedicled flaps used for plasty of head and neck defects

3.4.1 Percutaneous fat and cutaneous fascial flaps on a pedicle

a) The nasolabial flap is a true skin and fat flap, which is widely used for one-stage reconstruction of facial defects (nose and lip skin) and anterolateral oral cavity defects, including those with marginal resection of the mandible, floor of the mouth, hard palate, formed after surgery for neoplasms, as well as after various types of facial traumas and defects. This flap was first used in 1971 by H.A. Zarem for plasty of defects of the anterior parts of the oral cavity. The technique of flap formation is quite simple. The flap is cut out in the projection of the anterior surface of the cheek area. The width of the flap can vary depending on the state of turgor, elasticity of the facial skin and the severity of skin folds, on average from 2 to 3 cm, and in the elderly it reaches up to 5 cm. The flap length reaches up to 6 cm. In order to prevent a disruption of the blood supply, the flap should be cut thicker at the base than throughout the entire length. The flap itself, depending on its base, comes in two modifications: 1) a flap with the base at the corner of the mouth (Figure 28a). 2) a flap with a base at the nasal ramp and lower eyelid (Figure 28б).

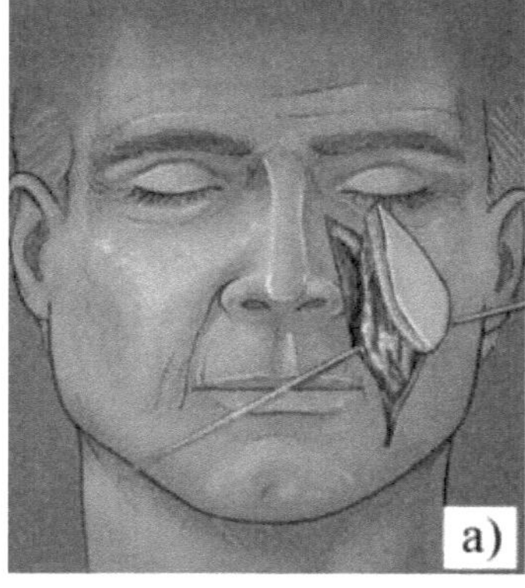

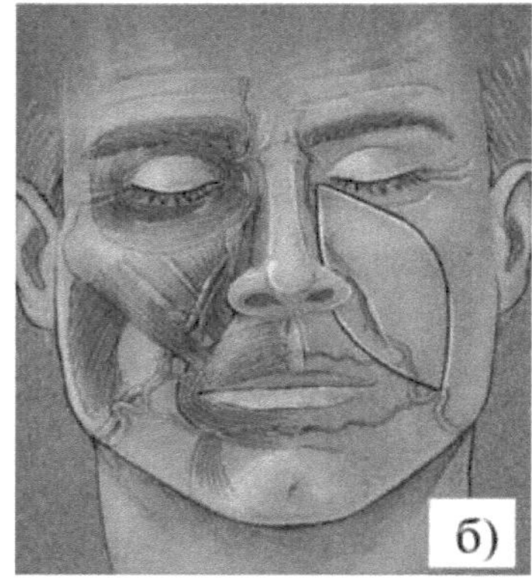

These modifications are of great clinical importance and are taken into account when reconstructing defects. The subcutaneous vascular network of the flap is supplied by branches of the facial artery. The nasolabial flap with the base at the lower eyelid and nasal ramp is fed by the *ophthalmic* artery (*a. ophtalmica*), which is a branch of the internal carotid artery system. The nasolabial graft with the base at the corner of the mouth is supplied with blood by the common facial artery (*a. fascialis communis), which is a branch of* the external carotid artery. The perforant arteries are mainly concentrated in the lower two thirds of the nasolabial fold and during the flap mobilisation it is necessary to take into account their inclusion in the flap pedicle in order to obtain a reliable vascular base. To replace defects of the anterior oral cavity area that extend beyond the midline, two nasolabial flaps can be cut from both sides at once. In this case, the stem is cut off from the base of the flap after 3 weeks with the closure of the orostomy.

The advantages of the nasolabial flap, regardless of the localisation of the feeding pedicle, include relative simplicity of the harvesting technique, acceptable cosmetic result, and good viability due to a rich blood supply, as it is the site of anastomosing of the terminal branches of the external and internal carotid arteries. Great mobility and sufficient length of the flap allow to form a duplicate for plasty of penetrating defects of the back and wing of the nose.

The main disadvantages of nasolabial flap plasty include the need to form delayed orostomies and the presence of a poorly expressed postoperative scar on the face, which prolongs the recovery period of patients. The use of the nasolabial flap in patients who have undergone radical lymphodissection on the same side of the neck is also discouraged, as it reduces the blood supply in the facial artery system.

The nasolabial flap was used in 30% of cases (32 flaps) of typical and combined plasty of facial, nasal, lip and oral cavity skin defects. Of these, cheiloplasty after excision of the lower lip cancer was performed in 14 (46.6%) cases. At the same time in 2 patients after complete removal of the lower lip the defect was plastically repaired with two nasolabial flaps. In 9 (30,0%) cases there was a cancer of the oral cavity, and in 2 patients with locally spread cancer of the mandibular alveolar process and in 2 patients with cancer of the cheek and lower lip mucosa the nasolabial flap was applied along with the BGM musculoskeletal flap, hyoid flap, cheek mucosa flap. In 4 (13.3%) cases the patients were operated on for skin cancer of the scutum and wing of the nose. Two patients (6.6%) had locally spread skin cancer of the zygomatic area, one patient (3.3%) had skin cancer of the left cheek area.

б) Cervical skin-fat, skin-fascial flap - this name means any skin-fat and skin-fascial flaps over the projection of the sternoclavicular-papillary muscle with or without inclusion of its fascia (a), flaps formed from the skin of the submandibular region with the base facing the mastoid process (b) and a flap from the posterior surface of the neck (c).

All these modifications of the cervical flap are supplied with blood by the musculoskeletal perforating branches of the underlying cervical muscles, which abundantly intertwine and anastomose to form a cervical vascular network; therefore, when preparing the flap, attention should be paid to a wide excision of the flap base, which guarantees adequate perfusion by as many perforating vessels as possible. The cervical flap can be used to close extensive defects of the oral cavity and the skin of the submandibular, cheek, parotid-cervical region. The flap should be cut out of the pre-irradiation zones. Particular attention should be paid to haemostasis, as there is a high risk of subcutaneous haematoma formation leading to flap necrosis. If the ratio of length to width is 2:1, the flap is well grafted, further increasing the length to width of the flap can increase the mobility of the flap, but the blood supply is disturbed, especially of its end fragments, which leads to necrosis. In patients with insufficient microcirculation, smokers, with concomitant diabetes mellitus, and received a preoperative course of radiation therapy there is a high risk of flap necrosis. In such cases, the cervical flap should be cut together with the underlying fragment of the subcutaneous muscle of the neck, which gives additional strength and volume, which can be used for 136

replace deeper defects in the head and neck area.

The advantages of the flap include the absence of the need for additional incisions with minimal increase in operative time. The disadvantages include relative thinness, mobility and vulnerability to necrotic complications.

We used cervical flaps in 7 (%) patients. Of these, there were 2 cases of typical defect plasty: in 1 patient for recurrent cancer of the auricle, and in 1 patient for locally advanced mucosal cancer of the mandibular alveolar outgrowth. The cervical flap was also used in five cases of combined defect plasty along with: a musculocutaneous flap on the pectoralis major muscle - 2 cases, a trapezius flap - 1 case, a flap from the saphenous muscle of the neck - 1 case, and a free split skin flap - 1 case.

в) **The frontal musculofascial flap is a** fairly well-studied flap and has long been widely used to replace skin defects of the face and nose. The first attempts to reconstruct nasal defects using the frontal flap were made in ancient India, where amputation of the nose was one of the methods of punishment. The method is known as "Indian" and is widely used by oncologists and plastic surgeons to this day.

The frontal flap consists of skin and subcutaneous tissue, cut together with the frontal fascia. This flap has a fairly rich blood circulation and is a good enough plastic material for replacing various non- and through (total) defects of the skin of the nose and perinasal region. The flap is supplied with blood by the frontal branches of the superficial temporal artery (*a. temporalis superior*) and the angular artery (*a. angularis*) from the facial artery system, which anastomose with each other to form a rich superficial (a) and deep (b) vascular network (Fig. 29).

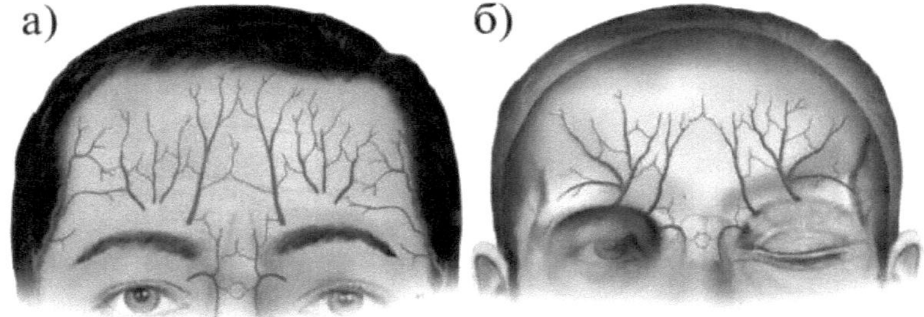

Figure 29. Superficial (a) and deep (b) vascular network of the frontal region

Depending on the location of the feeding pedicle, the flap has several modifications: medial, paramedial straight, paramedial oblique, medial, and gull wing flap (Figure 30).

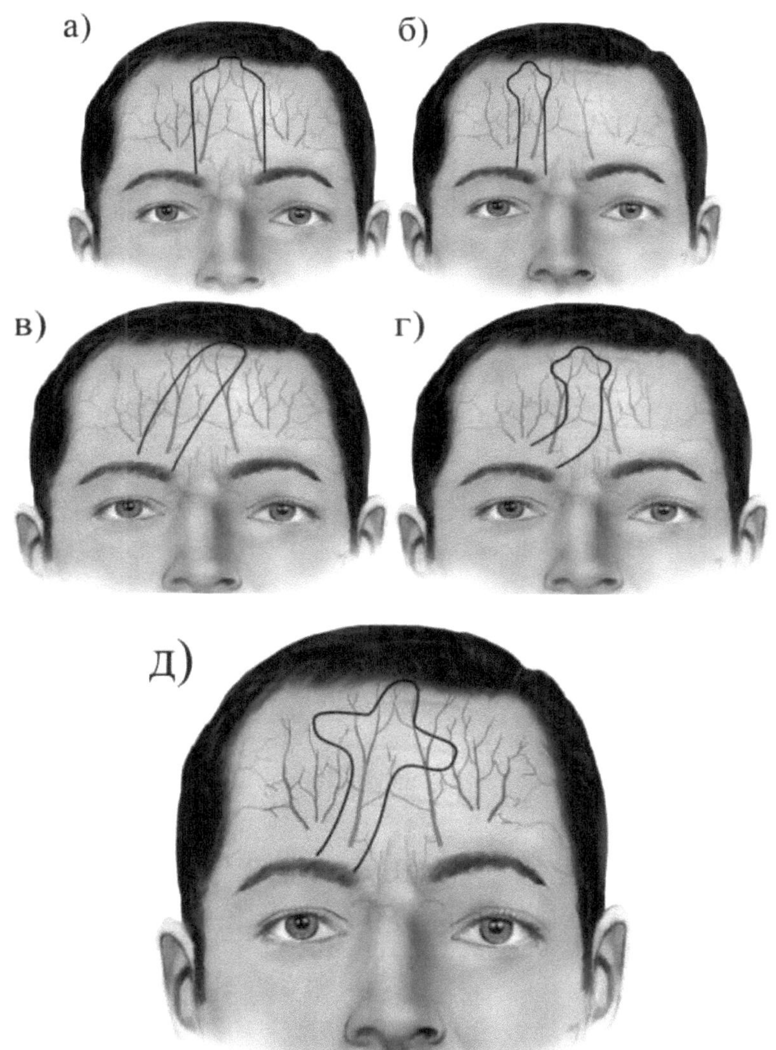

Figure 30. Modifications of the frontal flap: a) medial (Indian flap); b) paramedial vertical; c) paramedial oblique; d) midline; e) gull wing type flap

All of these modifications are sufficiently mobile and viable and can be applied to replace defects of the midface depending on their localisation. Another modification of the frontal flap is a cut on the arteriovenous bundle, which can be used to freely close subtotal skin defects of the eyelids, cheek and behind the ear. The high survivability of frontal flaps and the relative simplicity of the technique are expressed in the English-language literature by the term "lifeboat" and are recommended when the possibilities of previous reconstruction methods have been exhausted.

Disadvantages of the technique include postoperative scarring of the donor site causing a cosmetic deficit, as well as the two-stage nature of the method, as it is necessary to dissect the flap pedicle after 2-3 weeks of the main plastic surgery stage.

In our work, the frontal flap was used in 5 (3.8%) patients. Of these, in two cases after excision of locally advanced maxillary cancer, the flap served as a plastic material in replacing the skin defect of the maxillary region. Skin defects of the nasal ramus, cheek and parotid region were replaced in one case each.

г) **The submental islet flap is** a relatively new flap used in the reconstruction of head and neck defects (Martin et al., 1993) and numerous papers have shown the versatility of the flap in the reconstruction of defects of the face, neck and oropharynx.

This flap consists of a section of skin and subcutaneous fat of the submental region and the platysma, which is based on the submental artery *(a. submentalis)*, which is one of the terminal branches of the facial artery (Figure 31).

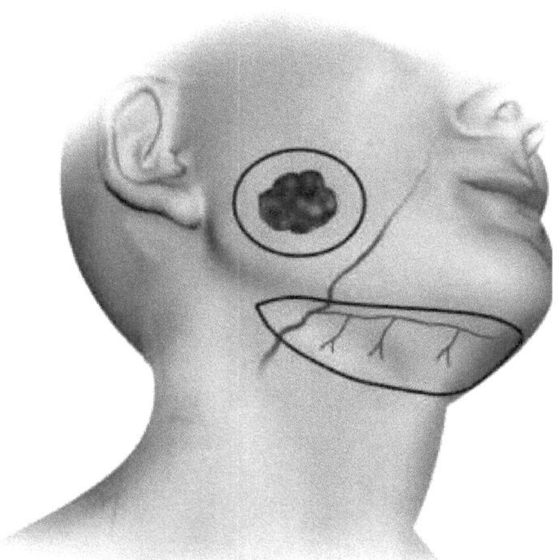

Figure 31. Landmarks and scheme of blood supply of the submental flap by branches of the chin artery

The advantages of this flap include (a) optimal mobility and a significant arc of rotation, allowing the flap to be moved at a sufficiently distant distance; (b) high viability; (c) minimal traumatic nature of the flap elevation process; (d) sufficient size (up to 84 cm^2) and volume of plastic material; (e) good functional and cosmetic results due to the commonality in skin colour and texture and (f) relatively short time required for flap excision.

However, the use of this flap has a number of disadvantages, in particular, the coincidence of the flap perfusion zone with the area of regional metastasis and difficulties in venous outflow. Also, when mobilising the flap, it is important to take into account the projection of the mandibular branch of the facial nerve, which passes close to the place of branching of the chin from the facial artery. Sometimes the massiveness of the flap requires some thinning of the flap thickness, which is achieved by cutting off the cutaneous fascial flap without including the subcutaneous neck muscle *(m. platysma).*

In our study, the submental flap was used in 4 (3.0%) patients. Of these, in three cases in typical plasty of defects for cancer of the red border of the lip, cheek mucosa and floor of the oral cavity. In one patient with locally advanced cancer of the cheek mucosa, combined plasty with the use of submental and trapezoidal musculocutaneous flaps was performed.

д) **The deltopectoral flap** was first used by Aymard in 1917 in the reconstruction of nasal defects, but gained popularity after its use by Bakamjian in 1965 and detailed description in the reconstruction of pharyngeal and oesophageal defects. The flap is a skin and fat flap from the projection of the antero-superior surface of the chest wall and deltoid muscle. This flap has long been used in reconstructive surgery of the head and neck and maxillofacial region and, along with the fasciocervico-pectoral flap, is one of the two frequently used flaps originating from the deltopectoral region.

Currently, the flap is very rarely used in the reconstruction of head and neck defects, particularly in cases where alternative methods of reconstruction are not available.

The flap belongs to the flaps with axial type of blood supply and is based on the perforating branches of the internal thoracic artery, which, coming out of the large pectoral muscle, penetrate the thoracic fascia at the rib and sternoclavicular junction and together with the accompanying veins of the same name go into the thickness of the subcutaneous fat, parallel to the clavicle at a distance of 10-12 cm almost to the middle of the length of the flap, then scattering, 142

form a network of small capillaries. The distal parts of the flap have chaotic blood supply. The base of the flap faces the sternum, laterally 2 cm from the edge of the sternum, where the flap pedicle is formed. The top of the flap is cut above the deltoid muscle, in the form of an arc connecting two horizontal incisions. Thus, it is possible to obtain a richly vascularised skin area 25-30 cm long and 6-8 cm wide, which can be used in combined plasty of through defects of the lower facial zone - lower lip, cheeks, lower lateral face and neck (Fig. 32).

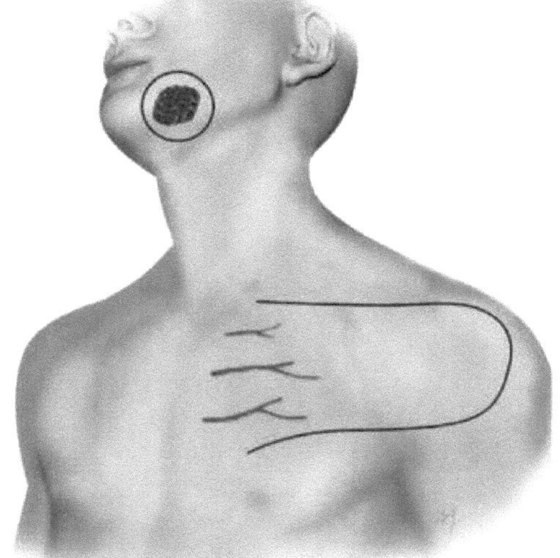

Figure 32. Circulation pattern and landmarks of the deltopectoral flap

In our study, deltopectoral flap was used in 2 (%) cases for locally
of advanced oral mucosal cancer. In one of them, an external lining of the oral cavity defect was created after surgery for locally advanced cancer of the cheek mucosa. In another patient, after excision of a tumour of the gingival mucosa of the mandibular alveolar process, a one-stage plasty of the defect was performed with a deltopectoral and musculocutaneous flap on the LGM.

e) Scalp flaps. The scalp is an area where it is possible to cut out "displaced" skin-fascial and skin-fat flaps for reconstruction of non-circumferential defects of the head. Due to the abundant blood supply of soft tissues of this area, which is provided by five paired arteries - superficial temporal, occipital and postauricular (from the external temporal artery system), supraorbital and supraclavicular - from the internal carotid artery system, which anastomose centrifugally, it is possible to cut flaps practically in any direction without disturbing the autonomy of their blood supply (Fig. 33).

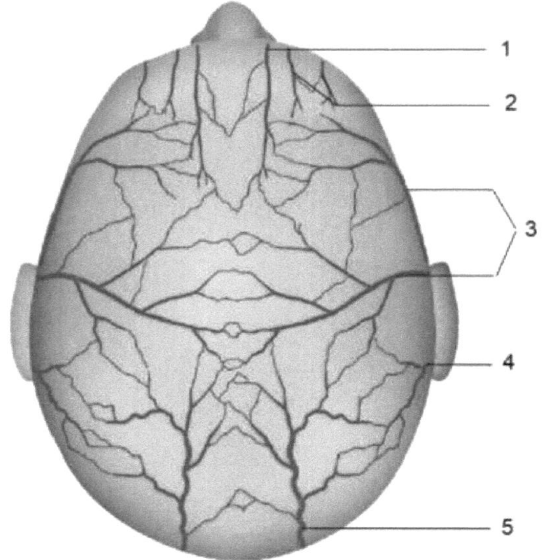

Figure 33. Vascular network of the scalp: 1) a. supratrochlearis superficialis; 2) a. supraorbitalis superficialis; 3) a. temporalis superior; 4) a. auricularis posterior; 5) a. occipitalis 144

In our work, scalp flaps were used in 6 cases in different modifications: temporal flap was used in 3 cases, of which 2 patients underwent plasty of category I defects for temporal and parietal skin cancer and 1 patient - for cancer of the right zygomatic region. Also in 3 cases, a displaced skin and fat flap from the occipital region (2 cases) and the parietal region (1 case) was used to close category I defects in locally spread skin cancer of the external ear.

3.4.2 MUSCULOSKELETAL FLAPS

The advent of vascularised dermal-muscular and free microsurgical flaps has reduced the popularity of regional dermal-fat and dermofascial flaps and significantly expanded the indications for operations with a reconstructive surgical stage. For the reconstruction of defects for locally disseminated head and neck cancer we did not limit ourselves to the use of only skin-fat and cutaneous fascial flaps. This is due to the fact that the massiveness of the mentioned flaps in most cases is not sufficient to fill deep deforming defects of facial tissues, in plasty of oral cavity defects - to resist the enzymatic activity of saliva, do not have a stabilised autonomous blood circulation.

Skin and muscle flaps on a vascular pedicle are of great importance in reconstructive and restorative surgeries for locally advanced head and neck cancer. The most important is the epithelial skin platform formed, which is brought to the skin or mucous membrane defect on a vascular base or base, the role of which is played by a skin tape, arteriovenous bundle or a strand of transverse striated muscle.

The blood supply of the skin and fat layer of the flap is provided by the perforating arteries coming from the main trunk of the underlying muscles and superficial cutaneous arteries coming directly from the main trunk, which bypass the muscles and are distributed in the underlying tissue. The working part of the flap can be formed along the entire length of the muscle or in the form of an island located on the distal part of the muscle. When lifting the flap, it is recommended to temporarily suture the distal ends of the skin and muscle to each other to prevent damage to the perforating vessels and preserve the natural unity of the skin-muscle block.

Our study included patients who underwent plasty of postoperative defects of the head and neck region with the following skin and muscle grafts:

1. Large pectoralis major muscle flap. It was first described by Ariyan in 1978 and, due to its versatility, remained the "workhorse" of head and neck defect reconstruction for several decades before the wide introduction of the free forearm flap into reconstructive oncological surgery [135, 137]. The flap has a pronounced axial blood supply, which is carried out by the brachial pectoral artery, which originates from the axillary artery (1-3 branches), penetrating the internal fascia of the pectoralis major muscle, obliquely heading to the sternum. The skin area above the muscle is supplied with blood by the perforating arteries that run vertically through the muscle and require special care during flap harvesting (Figure 34).

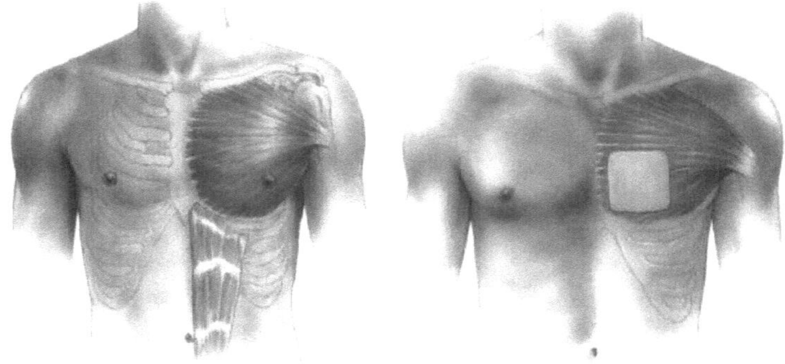

Figure 34. Large pectoral muscle - approximate flap dimensions

According to the structure of the feeding pedicle, the flap of the pectoralis major muscle is represented by several modifications (Figure 35).

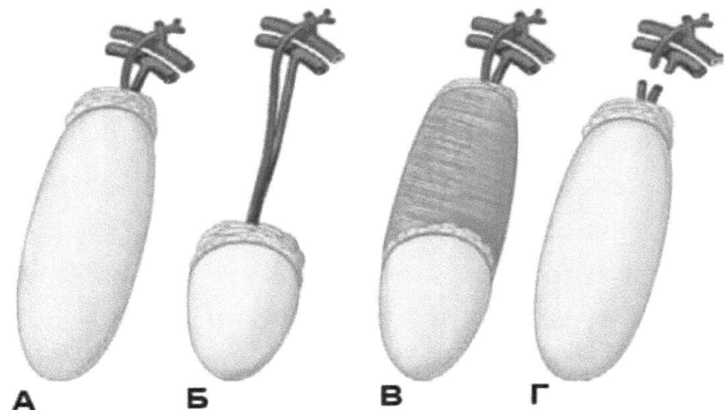

*Figure 35. Variants of the musculocutaneous flap on the
pectoralis major muscle*

The modification (Figure 35 A) is used for plasty of extensive defects of the head and neck, laryngo- and pharyngostoma [116, 136]. It is a flap with a full-layer pedicle in which the size of the skin-fat pad corresponds to the size of the underlying muscle. The end section closes the defect of the facial mucosa, the base can cover the vascular bundle and defects of the neck tissues along the course of the base. Another modification is the true islet flap, which is formed according to the size of the defect in the distal end of the pectoral muscle and is brought to the defect on the vascular pedicle (Figure 35-B). When mobilising this type of flap, the sternoacromial vessels should be carefully isolated all the way to their penetration into the muscle. The third modification, most commonly used, is based on a muscle pedicle that is larger than the dermal fat island (Figure 35-B). In this modification, the repair is performed at the expense of the end fragment of the flap, and the muscle base is brought to the defect through a subcutaneous tunnel, in which it is inconspicuous, but can serve to cover the main vessels of the neck. Finally, a fourth modification of the flap is cut out in proportion to the defect with cutting off the feeding vessels for microsurgical anastomosis with the recipient vessels of the neck (Figure 35-G).

The advantages of this flap include the following characteristics: The flap is remote from the radiation areas during the treatment of head and neck cancer. The technical harvesting of the flap is not very difficult, and two teams of surgeons can participate simultaneously to reduce operative time. The massiveness of the soft tissues of the flap allows its application as an ideal graft in the reconstruction of extensive through and combined defects of the oral cavity and oropharynx, to fill the tissue deficit of the named areas. The flap adapts well to the defect and is ideal for one-stage reconstruction of head and neck defects. The abundant blood circulation of the flap makes it possible to form a single skin and fat islet of almost the entire surface of the large pectoral muscle or two skin islets on a single pedicle, which can be used to form an inner and outer lining to close through defects of the oral cavity. The flap's arc of rotation and mobility are sufficient to close most oropharyngeal and lateral neck defects. The donor defect usually heals by primary tension and the postoperative scar remains in the anterior chest wall, which is usually covered by clothing.

The disadvantages of the flap include excessive massiveness in the reconstruction of shallow defects of the face and oral cavity, especially in women with large mammary glands, and, therefore, it should be used as a pure-muscular flap in combination with a split skin graft. In the reconstruction of defects of the oral cavity and oropharynx it tends to be rejected due to the force of attraction, which leads to divergence of the suture line in the upper parts of the wound. The mobility of the flap is limited when reconstructing the defects of the upper parts of the face and upper jaw. Symmetry of the trunk in the donor site is disturbed and causes aesthetic discomfort, especially in women. The function of the shoulder is compromised due to disruption of the integrity of the pectoralis major muscle. The skin distal to the flap is somewhat unstable in most cases. A musculoskeletal flap with the inclusion of a fragment of the IV-V rib can be used in the reconstruction of mandibular defects, but it is not recommended because of the insufficient strength of the rib and its poor blood supply.

In the study, 37 (34.2%) patients with head and neck cancer were used skin-muscular flaps on the pectoralis major muscle for defect reconstruction. Of these, 33 (89.2%) patients used the flap to replace defects of the oral cavity mucosa and tongue, of which 3 (8.1%) cases were combined with dermofascial flaps (dermofascial nasolabial and cervical flaps). Also, in 1 case, the flap was applied with the segment of the V rib in combination with a dermuscular subclavian and dermofascial nasolabial flap. In the remaining 4 (10.2%) patients, this flap was used for facial defects - 3 cases and lip defects - 1 case.

2. Sternoclavicular-papillary flap (SCFL) - since the first description of the flap by N. Owens in 1955, this flap is considered the most rarely used plastic material. The musculocutaneous sternoclavicular-papillary flap is formed on the projection of the muscle of the same name and includes the skin with subcutaneous fatty tissue and the entire muscle itself or only one of its legs. Depending on the size of the defect, the skin of the flap can be mobilised along the entire length of the muscle or in the form of an islet.

The muscle itself has a segmental blood supply from several sources: the upper third from the occipital artery, the middle third from the superior thyroid and external carotid artery, and the lower third is variable and receives blood from the thyroid trunk, supra scapular and transverse cervical arteries.

Two modifications of the flap are known: the first one with the base facing upwards, which is ideal for plasty of defects of the parotid region of the lower face after parotidectomy, and the anterior parts of the oral cavity. The second modification is with a downward-facing base, which can be used to close gaping defects of the pharynx and the cervical oesophagus (Figure 36).

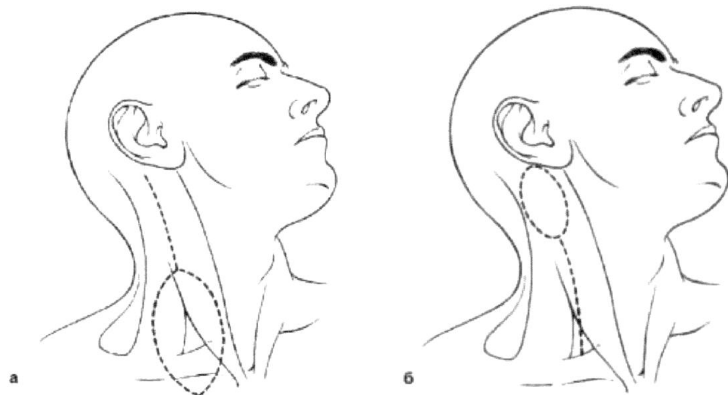

Figure 36. Schematic of cutting a modification of a complex musculocutaneous sternoclavicular-papillary flap: a) base facing upwards, b) base facing downwards

The disadvantages of the flap include a high incidence of complications in the form of complete or partial necrosis of the skin flap site, and its use in patients who undergo bilateral fascial-futlar surgery
excision of the neck fibres, often inappropriate.
We have reconstructed postoperative defects with this flap in 12 patients. Of them, defects of the 1st group after excision of recurrent skin tumour of temporal and behind-the-ear region - 2 patients, defects of the 2nd group - in 10 patients with cancer of oral cavity organs (defects of the 3rd group): which were located in the lower jaw - 4, tongue - 3, cheek mucosa and floor of the mouth - 1 patient each. It should be noted that in 1

patient the sternoclavicular-papillary flap was used in combination with the sternal hyoid flap. Sternal hyoid flap **(SHF)** - Another musculoskeletal flap cut on the anterior surface of the neck is a flap on the anterior long muscles of the neck - the sternal hyoid flap (SHF). This flap was first used by Wang et al. (1986) to replace defects of the oral cavity. The working area of the flap is formed by a skin-fat islet cut out in proportion to the defect above the jugular notch of the sternum, which is attached to the sterno- hyoid muscle, which is the base. The muscle is cut off from the sternum and mobilised up to the place of its attachment to the hyoid bone and raised in a single block with the skin, as a result we get a mobile graft, which can be easily brought to the defects of the oral cavity and lateral walls of the oropharynx (Fig. 37).

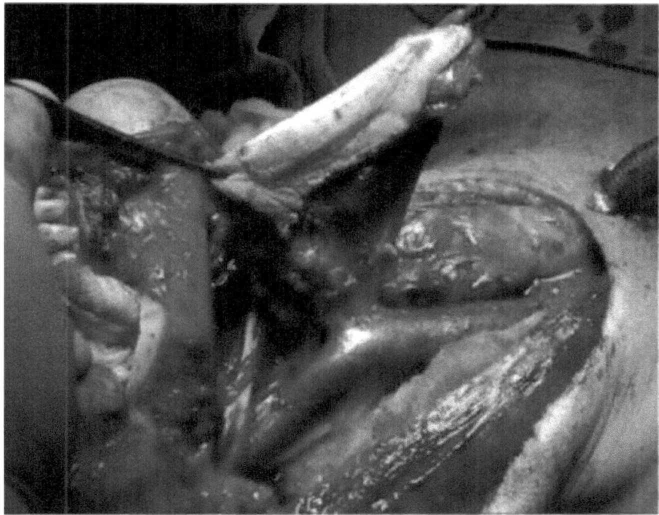

Figure 37. Dermusculoskeletal flap on the sternothoracolumbar muscles of the neck

The blood supply to the muscle is provided by the superior and inferior thyroid arteries, but during flap dissection, branches of the inferior thyroid artery are excised, and the dominant role in providing blood flow 152

of the flap is led to the hyoid branches of the superior thyroid artery. For reliable blood supply of the flap, it is possible to cut a skin-fat pad on both muscles at once, in which case capillary networks abundantly intertwine and anastomose with each other. The skin-fat flap fragment is formed with a diameter of about 5 cm. The muscle itself is very thin and pliable, and such a flap is convenient to use for plasty of small defects of the anterior parts of the oral cavity and after half resections of the tongue.

We present the results of reconstruction of defects of groups 2 and 3 in 12 patients. Of these, there were 6 cases of mucosal cancer of the mandibular alveolar process, 3 cases of cheek mucosal cancer, 2 cases of mucosal cancer of the floor of the oral cavity, and 1 case of tongue cancer.

3. Percutaneous muscle flap based on the saphenous muscle (platysma) (PL). The principles of the first use of a dermuscular flap based on the subcutaneous muscle of the neck was first described by the Austrian surgeon Robert Gersuny (1887). He used this graft to reconstruct a through cheek defect. Later, Futrell et al. (1978) gave a complete description and characterisation of the islet flap based on the saphenous muscle of the neck used for plasty of oral cavity defects.

The platysma is a paired muscle lying just under the skin, which starts at the clavicle, then runs up the anterior and lateral surface of the neck, ends slightly above the edge of the lower jaw and is intertwined with the fibres of the mimic muscles. Its blood supply is provided by branches of the facial, upper thyroid and superficial artery of the neck. There are three modifications of the flap according to the basins of the blood supplying vessels: 1) on the upper base - from the basin of the submandibular branch of the facial artery, 2) on the lower base

- supplied by the transverse cervical artery, and 3) on the posterior base - supplied by branches of the occipital and posterior auricular arteries.

We used this flap in 3 cases to replace defects of group 4. In 2 patients with laryngeal cancer the flap based on the subcutaneous muscle of the neck was used to repair the laryngostomy defect, in 1 patient the defect of the anterior surface of the cervical trachea was replaced.

4. Trapezoidal flap (TFL). This flap is ideal for reconstructing defects of the posterior surface of the neck, and the length of the muscle pedicle and the thickness of the vascular trunk allow the flap to be rotated 180 degrees and brought to various defects of the parotid-cervical, temporal, anterior surface of the neck and mandible. The trapezius muscle and the skin above it are supplied with blood mainly by superficial and deep branches of the transverse neck artery (*a. cervicalis transversus*) and *occipital* artery (*a.* occipitalis).

The flap on the trapezius muscle has several modifications: a flap on a musculoskeletal, muscular only and vascular pedicle, which can be cut to the entire length of the muscle. One of the disadvantages of this flap is the need to change the patient's position on the operating table, which somewhat lengthens the operation time and makes it uncomfortable for surgeons. This need to change the patient's position can be eliminated by placing the patient on the side opposite to the side where the flap is taken.

The trapezoidal flap was used in 1 case to replace a parotid defect for recurrent parietal skin cancer (a clinical example is given in Chapter 3). The comparative characteristics of patients by the categories of defects formed in the main, control, and total cohort of patients are shown in Table 20.

Table 20. - Comparative characterisation of patients by

categories of defects formed in the main, control groups and the total cohort of patients

Category of defects	Main group		Control group		Total		P
I	24	22,2%	12	19,7%	36	21,3%	*0.698*
II	70	64,8%	46	75,4%	116	68,6%	*0.154*
III	10	9,3%	3	4,9%	14	8,3%	*0.474*
IV	4	3,7%	0	0%	3	2,4%	-
Total	108	100%	61	100%	169	100%	

Note: *p* - statistical significance of the difference between the indicators of the main and control groups (by Pearson's $\%^2$ criterion).

In general, the same regularity in the distribution of defects among patients in the main and control groups can be traced. The highest frequency of defects formed in all groups is category II defects - 64.8% and 75.4%, respectively. They are followed in frequency by category I defects - 22.2% and 19.7%. Category III defects, which are represented by penetrating defects of mucous membranes, muscles and bones communicating with the skin surface over a large length, were formed relatively less frequently (9.3% and 4.9%, respectively). Defects of group IV by frequency of occurrence in the main group accounted for the smallest number of observations - 3.7%, and there were none in the control group. Among the patients of the main group (n = 108) 103 (95,4%) underwent reconstruction with skin-fat, skin-muscular and other flaps simultaneously with the main volume of the operation on tumour removal, only 5 (4,6%) patients underwent the reconstructive stage in a delayed order, of which 2 patients - because of the recurrence of the tumour of the oral cavity organs after complex treatment, and 3 - after a six-month recurrence-free period. In the control group 53 (86,9%) patients after the tumour excision stage underwent only simple stitching of the defect edges, and 8 (13,1%) underwent minimal volume - defect plasty with local tissues - 4 cases, and in other 4 cases - with a free split skin graft (Table 21).

Table 21. - Types and frequency of surgical interventions in the studied groups

Timing and type of reconstruction	Main group		Control group		Total	
One-stage flap plasty	103	95,4%	-	-	103	95,4%
Deferred patchwork	5	4,6%	-	-	5	4,6%
Suturing the wound edges	-	-	53	86,9%	53	86,9%
Local tissue grafting	-	-	4	6,5%	4	6,5%
No plastics.	-	-	4	6,5%	4	6,5%
Total	108	100%	61	100%	169	100%

When analysing the frequency of surgical interventions (Table 21), it can be seen that in the main group, 95.4% of patients underwent one-stage reconstructive interventions with the use of certain flaps and only in 5 (4.6%) cases the plastic surgery was delayed. In the control group the reconstructive stage was minimised by limiting the stitching of the postoperative wound edges - 86.9%, local tissues - 6.5%, and in 6.5% of cases the plastic was not performed at all.

CHAPTER 4

RESULTS OF HEAD AND NECK DEFECT PLASTY, THEIR IMPACT ON QUALITY OF LIFE PARAMETERS AND LONG-TERM RESULTS

4.1. Evaluation of immediate and near-term results of defect reconstruction. Analysis of postoperative complications

As mentioned above, reconstruction of head and neck defects reached its heyday with the invention and introduction into clinical practice of methods of taking vascularised skin-fat and skin-muscle flaps.

An extensive tissue defect is defined as a lack of tissue following excision of a tumour involving several adjacent anatomical regions or organs. Such defects are usually formed after radical extended operations for locally disseminated tumours and, as a rule, they cannot be eliminated by simple suturing of the wound edges and require mandatory reconstructive replacement. Consequently, we strictly adhere to the opinion about the necessity of one-stage plasty of postoperative defects, as it allows to perform surgery with radicalism and shortens the period of rehabilitation of patients.

4.1.1 Results of reconstruction of
skull vault
and neck skin defects

Squamous cell skin cancer of the scalp has an aggressive course and more often affects all layers of the skin, sprouting up to the bones of the skull vault. Depending on the type of the formed defects, we used almost the whole arsenal of available skin-fat, skin-muscle flaps and free skin grafts. According to the results of our observations in the studied area the most acceptable is plasty with a free skin graft, which is usually taken with a dermatome from such donor areas as the anterior surface of the shoulder or thigh. This technique is easy to perform, safe and less damaging to the donor area.

Exceptions are cases when free split skin is transplanted onto a bone devoid of periosteum, which is fraught with complications in the form of flap non-union and its necrosis, which nullifies the expected result. In these cases, we used skin-fascial and skin-muscular flaps on a pedicle, which were cut from the skin areas bordering the defect, and the donor defect of the skull vault was closed with a free skin flap. Due to the abundant blood supply of the cranial vault skin, it is possible to cut out cutaneous fascial flaps in any direction and over long distances. The scalp defect plasty was performed in 12 patients with squamous cell cancer, T2N0M0-T4N1M0. The number of flaps used is shown in Table 22.

Table 22. - Distribution of patients depending on the applied flaps and localisation of the defect

Flap	Skull vault defects
Free split skin flap	5
Cervical	1
Sternoclavicular-papillary.	2
Trapezoidal	1
BGM	1
Other flaps	5
Flap combination	4 (26,6%)
Total	15 (100%)

Thus, 12 patients underwent plastic surgeries using 15 different flaps, of which 4 had combined plastic surgeries where more than one flap was used. These methods of defect replacement are successful and, in our opinion, worthy of application in clinical practice.

To demonstrate the possibilities of surgical treatment of cranial vault squamous cell carcinoma, we present the following clinical example:

Clinical example. *Patient M.K., 75 years old, a pensioner (former driver), has been registered at the RONC since 01.01.1991 with the diagnosis "Primary multiple skin cancer of the head and neck". He applied on 08.01.2014 with complaints about the presence of a tumour of the right temporal region, shooting pains of constant character with irradiation to the neck and occiput. From anamnesis it was found out that the appearance of the tumour was two years old, the patient underwent a non-radical surgery in a rural polyclinic at the place of residence. Since the appearance of the tumour at the operation site, the patient had been engaged in "self-treatment", heat therapy, etc. The patient had a history of a two-year old tumour.*

procedures and ointment dressings - without effect, which led to rapid growth of the tumour and increase of the above symptoms. On examination, there is an exophytic tumour on the skin of the right temporoparietal region, measuring 7.0xb.0 cm, painful, bleeding,   not displaceable,

infiltrating the underlying tissues and the right auricle. There is no evidence of enlargement of regional lymph nodes and tumour penetration into the adjacent bones of the skull vault according to the CT scan of the head dated 04.01.2014. After histological verification of the diagnosis (squamous cell cancer with keratinisation No.216 dated 08.01.2014 the patient received radiation therapy from 16.01.2014 to 29.01.2014. ROD - 3 Gy / SOD - 30 Gy. On 19.02.2014 he was hospitalised in the surgical department #3 (medical history #838). After examination and correction of concomitant diseases the patient with the diagnosis of right temporoparietal tumour recurrence

T4N0M0 on 27.02.2014 underwent a combined operation (№62) in the scope of "Excision of skin tumour of the right temporo-occipital region with resection of the upper third of the auricle. Plasty of the defect with a skin-fat cervical flap". Primary wound healing. Histological report №2630 from 27.02.2014 squamous cell keratinising cancer G1, with invasion of all skin layers and moderate treatment pathomorphosis. The patient was discharged on the 12th day after surgery.

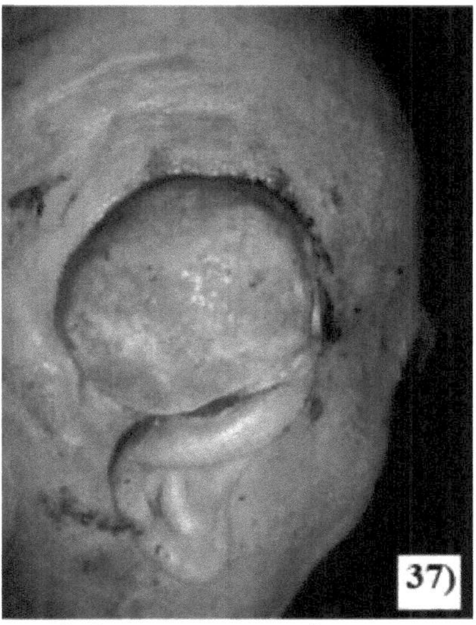

Figure 37. Temporal skin cancer with extension into the auricle

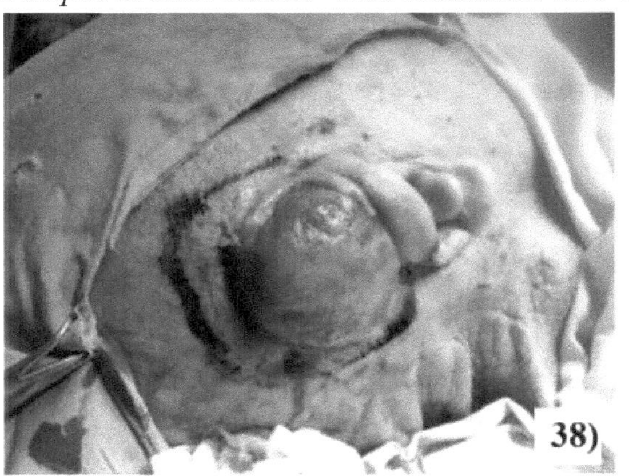

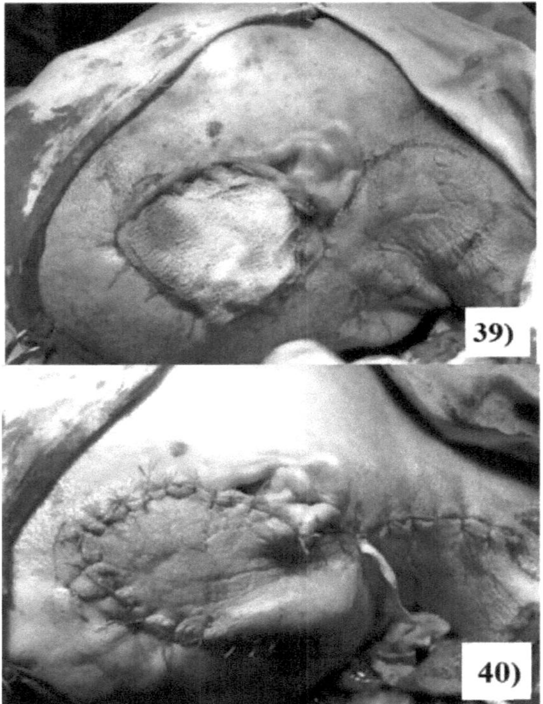

Figure 39. Marking of the excised loxcutis commensurate with the defect after tumour excision

Figure 40. The flap is brought up and sutured to the defect

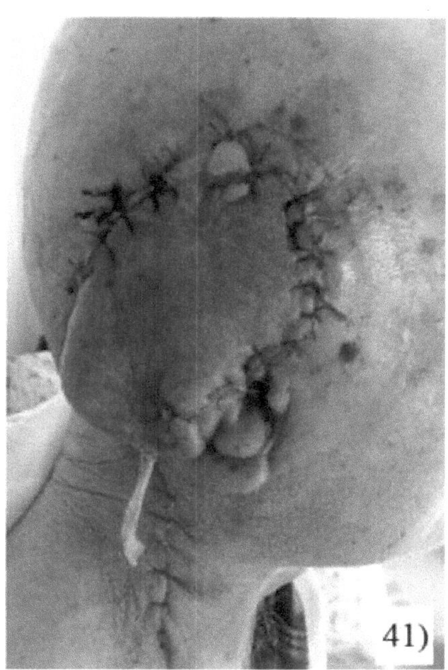

Figure 41. View of the flap on the second day after surgery. There is insignificant swelling of the flap

Two years later, on 02.02.2016, the patient presented with a new recurrence of the tumour and a new nidus on the skin of the right temporal region 2.5x3.0 cm. On examination at the site of the previous surgery, a recurrent tumour of 8.0x7.0 cm. dense, soldered conglomerate, painful on palpation with bleeding surface was noted. Radiation therapy was recommended to the patient by the decision of the consilium. From 10.10.2016 to 28.10.2016 the patient underwent radiotherapy ROD - 3 Gy/C0D - 45 Gy.

On 04.11.2016, he was hospitalised in the Department of General Otology (hospital #5656) for a second operation. Ultrasound examination of the neck (06.10.2016) revealed a metastatic cervical lymph node enlarged up to 1.5 cm in the upper third on the right side, which forms a single conglomerate with the tumour. According to CT examination

147

163 *there were no signs of involvement of the cranial bones. After examination by a therapist and cardiologist, the patient was diagnosed with cardiovascular system: ischaemic heart disease, focal cardiosclerosis, arterial hypertension of the I degree, risk 4. Gastrointestinal tract organs: biliary dyskinesia, hepatosis of II degree, reactive pancreatitis. Urinary system organs - left kidney cyst, chronic pyelonephritis, prostate adenoma (Figure 42).*

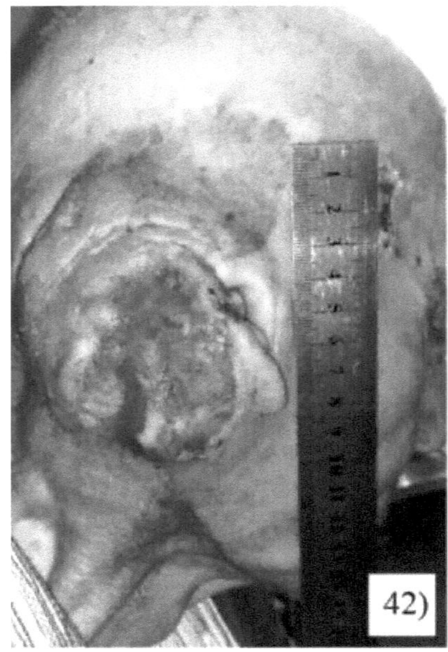

Figure 42. Recurrent tumour of the right behind-the-ear region

The patient underwent a repeat operation (#394) "Excision of recurrent tumour of the right behind-the-ear region on 18.11.2016. Fascial-futlar excision of the neck fibre on the right side, upper variant. Plasty of the defect with a skin-muscular flap with inclusion of the right trapezius muscle and a skin-fascial cervical flap". The duration of the operation was 200 minutes. The wound healing is primary. The sutures were removed on the 10th-11th day. Pathohistological report №9284 dated 18.11.2016 - squamous cell keratinising carcinoma G2,

148

with invasion into adjacent soft tissues. The tumour was removed within healthy tissues. The patient was discharged on the 17th day, the follow-up period was 5 years and 4 months (Figures 43 - 47).

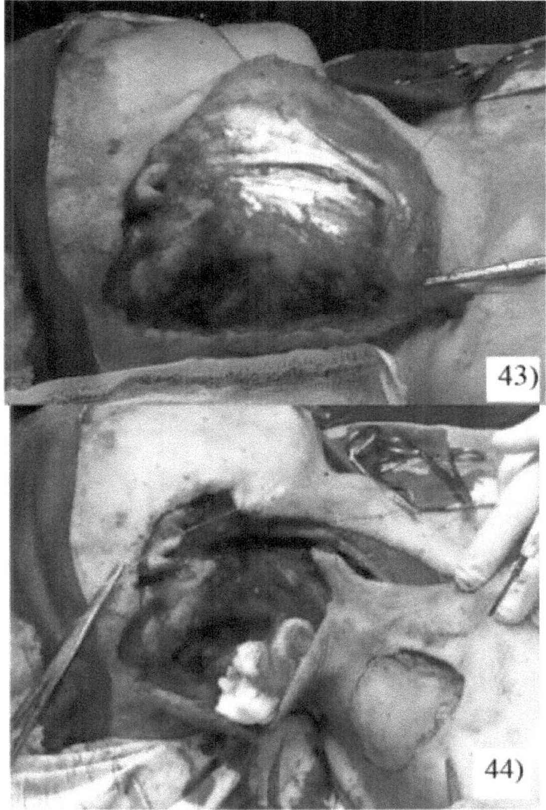

Figure 43. Stage of surgery - tumour removed together with the cervical fibre
Figure 44. Marking of the skin flap site

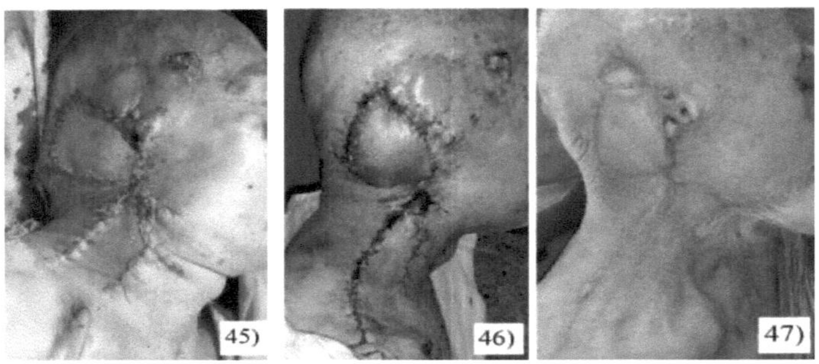

Figure 45. Final view of the patient after surgery
Figure 46. View of the flap on the fourth day after surgery
Figure 47. Result of plasty 3 months after surgery

4.1.2 Results of plastic surgery of facial defects

We included non-cutaneous skin defects of the parotid, zygomatic, cheek, nose, lips, and chin area as facial skin defects. All these localisations were combined into one group due to the common anatomical features of reconstructive techniques and the plastic material used. Immediately before surgery in the facial region it is necessary to take into account the nature and volume of tissues removed with the tumour, pathomorphological characteristics, stages of the tumour process. The main goal of reconstruction is considered to be the achievement of maximum functional and cosmetic results with a mandatory focus on the parameters of patients' quality of life.

A decaying tumour on the face with a foul-smelling odour is often a strong depressive factor leading to psychosocial discomfort for the patient, and sometimes 166

suicidal behaviour. Such patients often cannot fully communicate with the people around them and even with their family members, which leads to the development of the stigma of inferiority and severe stress in the patient. All this gives us a reason to decide on one-stage plasty of the defects. To restore facial defects, we used the following skin-fascial and skin-muscular flaps, which are summarised in Table 23.

Table 23. - Types of flaps used for plasty of facial defects

Localisation of the defect/ Flap	Lips	Periradicular ar-	Cheekbone	oblast	.	Nose	Cheek	Total
BGM	1	2	-	-		-	-	3
Temennoi	-	1	-	-		-	-	1
Posterior	-	2	-	-		-	-	2
Cervical	-	1	1	-		-	-	2
Nasolabial	14	-	2	-		4	1	21
Frontal	-	1	-	1		1	1	4
Loose leather	-	1	1	1		-	-	3
Local tissues	-	2	1	1		-	1	5
Total	15	10	5	3		5	3	41

Thus, the most frequent plasty of lip defects was performed - 15 operations (34.1%), and in the overwhelming majority (14 cases) a skin-fat, skin-fascial nasolabial flap was used independently, and only in 1 case - a skin-muscular flap on the pectoralis major muscle. Less frequently, in 10 (24.3%) observations, reconstructive surgery was performed for defects of the skin and soft tissues of the periocervical region, where the we combined the defects formed at excision of skin cancer of the auricle and behind the ear region, as well as at metastases of cranial vault skin cancer to the lymph nodes of the parotid salivary gland, in which parotidectomy is performed with/without preserving the branches of the facial nerve, where we used a skin-muscular flap of the BGM - in 2 cases and various types of skin-fat and skin-fascial flaps - in 8 cases. We consider the plasty of the defects of the zygomatic and frontal temporal region to be no less effective, which took place in 5 and 3 cases, respectively, which were replaced with skin-fat and skin-fascial flaps from the border regions. In the third place by frequency of observations is skin cancer of different subunits of the nose - in 5 (12,2%) cases, and replacement of defects in 4 of them was performed with the help of a nasolabial flap. The least frequent defects were formed in the cheek area, which took place in 3 (7.3%) cases, which were replaced with skin-fat and skin-fascial flaps from adjacent areas. Here are some examples from clinical observations.

Patient N., 66 years old, (medical history No. 2969) on 23.05.2017 complained of a skin tumour of the left auricle, pain, bleeding, weakness, malaise. From the anamnesis - he has been registered at the RONC since 22.07.2014. The first operation was performed in June 2014 in the volume of excision of the skin tumour of the behind-the-ear region and suturing of the wound edges. Histological report (#4426) from 2014. - Squamous cell carcinoma with a tendency to keratinisation. In 2016, the patient received a full course of adjuvant radiotherapy SOD - 72 Gy. Subsequently, the patient did not seek medical attention.

When the patient came back to the above-mentioned complaints, the examination revealed a recurrent skin tumour of the left behind-the-ear region 3.0 x 2.0 cm in diameter, with a dirty plaque, painful on palpation, with little displacement. Regional lymph nodes are not enlarged. The patient had typical concomitant diseases, in particular, CHD, arterial hypertension of II degree, risk III, atherosclerosis of cerebral vessels, chronic bronchitis, cholecystitis.

Under general endotracheal anaesthesia on 01.06.2017, the patient underwent surgery (#182) in the scope of excision of a recurrent skin tumour of the left auricle with resection of the auricle. The plasty of the formed defect was performed with a skin-fat cervical flap. The postoperative period proceeded without peculiarities. The flap engraftment and wound healing were primary. Pathohistological diagnosis #1110 dated 01.06.2017 "Expressed healing pathomorphosis with the presence of multinucleated foreign cells". Sutures were removed on the 7th-8th day after surgery. The duration of follow-up was 58 months (Figures 48 to 50).

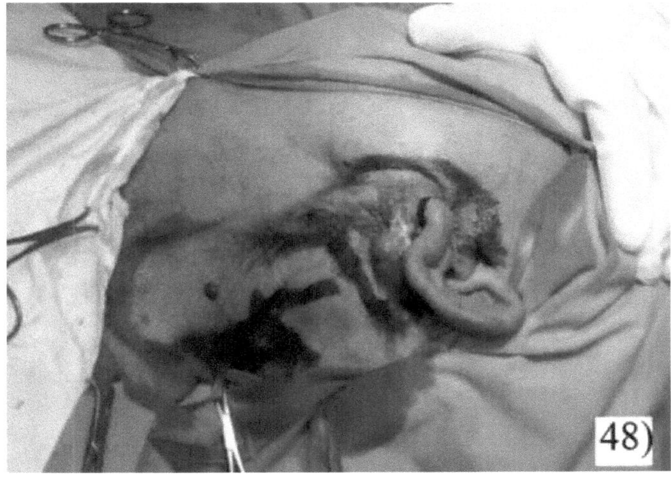

Figure 48. - Locally advanced recurrent T4N0M0 skin cancer of the behind-the-ear region, postoperative status 2014 and HCT 2016, patient 66 years old.   (case   history   #2969), preoperative mark-up

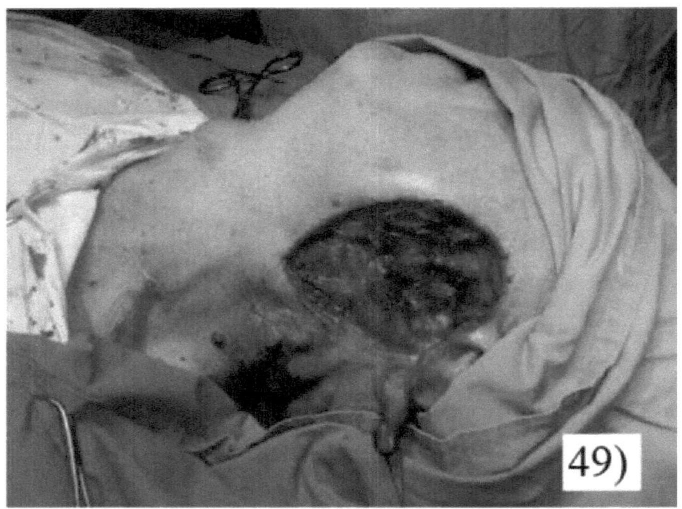

Figure 49. - Postoperative defect formed

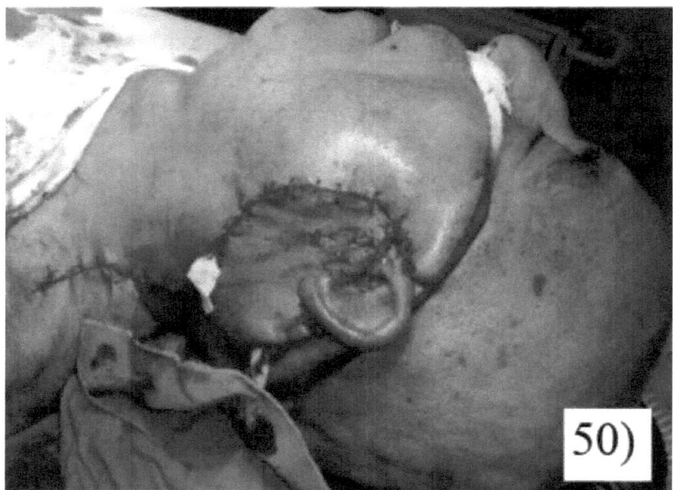

Figure 50. Defect replaced with a dermofascial cervical flap on a vertical pedicle

This clinical observation shows the efficacy of reconstructive and restorative surgery.
for recurrent behind-the-ear tumour.

4.1.3 Reconstruction of oral defects

Cancer of the oral cavity occupies the second place in the morbidity structure of head and neck tumours, and has the most unfavourable course and outcome. This is due to the complexity of the anatomical structure of the oral cavity as the beginning of the aerodigestive tract and the functions of this area. Unfortunately, the percentage of neglect of locally advanced cases of oral cancer in our country, as well as in all developing countries remains stably high, and makes up to 75-80%. This is due to low public awareness and lack of cancer vigilance among primary care doctors, failure to observe the principles of basic oral hygiene, lack of screening programmes and measures for early detection of precancerous diseases and oral cancer. In addition to the above factors, a common bad habit among the male population - smokeless tobacco smoking or use of nasvay (betel) and insufficient awareness of patients about the seriousness of this oncopathology and the possibilities of the oncological service and the achievements of modern oncology and head and neck surgery - are of great importance. Also in recent years, the diagnosis of cancer of the oral cavity and nasopharynx has become relatively more frequent in patients of relatively young age - 25-35 years old, who have no history of bad habits, which gives the preconditions to think about a possible viral carcinogenesis.

Volumetric surgeries on the oral cavity organs result in permanent complex defects that lead to impairment of vital body functions, in particular speech, chewing, swallowing and breathing, which are disabling factors and a reason for patients to refuse the proposed surgical intervention.

Tumour excision and at the same time large volumes of soft tissues of the oral cavity with resection of the jaw bones lead to persistent, irreversible functional and cosmetic changes, which subsequently lead to excessive psycho-emotional stress with decreased self-esteem of patients, deep irreversible depression up to suicidal outcomes [50].

In this regard, we believe that reconstruction and repair of extensive defects should be performed simultaneously at the stage of the main operation for removal of the primary tumour. This, in turn, makes it possible to expand the indications for surgery and the volume of excised tissues of the oral cavity and contributes to the achievement of maximum radicalism. Correctly performed reconstructive and restorative surgery even in neglected patients for some time relieves unfavourable symptoms of the disease (pain, odour, discomfort) and improves their quality of life, thus providing patients with their everyday relative comfort and enabling them to socially integrate.

In our study, out of the total cohort, 113 (66.9%) patients in the main (67) and control (46) groups developed some form of oral defects of different complexity categories (Table 24).

Table 24. - Frequency of defects by category in the main and control groups

Category of defect	Main group	Control group	Total
Category I	24	12	36 (21,3%)
	p = 0.151		
II category	70	46	116(68,6%)
	p = 0.014		
III category	11	3	14 (8,3%)
	p = 0.340		
IV category	3	-	3 (1,8%)
Total	67 (59,3%)	46 (40,7%)	169 (100%)
	p = 0.077		

Note: p - statistical significance of the difference between the indicators of the main and control groups (by Pearson's $\%^2$ criterion).

The frequency of defects formed according to excision of tumours of different organs and tissues is shown in Table 25.

Table 25. - Frequency of defects formed depending on tumour localisation

The defects are due to the removal of a tumour	Main group n, (%)	Control group n, (%)	Total n, (%)	P x²
Face, head and neck skin	24	12	36	0.698
Alv. detachment of the n/maxilla.	25	11	36	0.436
Cheek mucosa	23	2	24	0.004
Language	7	16	23	<0,001
The red border of the lips	14	1	15	0.028
Upper jaw	1	13	13	<0,001
The floor of the mouth	9	2	11	0.340
Alv. c/ jaw.	2	4	6	0.113
Larynx	2	-	2	-
of the thyroid gland	1	-	1	-
Total	108 (100%)	61 (100%)	169 (100%)	

Note: p - statistical significance of the difference between the indicators of the main and control groups (by Pearson's $\%^2$ criterion).

It was found that defects are most often formed by excision of tumours of the skin of the head and neck, the alveolar process of the mandible and the cheek mucosa, then the tongue, lips, upper jaw, floor of the oral cavity and the alveolar process of the upper jaw. We used the following types of flaps to restore defects of the mucous membrane and oral organs (Table 26).

Table 26. - Frequency of graft use depending on the localisation of oral cavity defects

^\Localisation \ defect Scraps		Alv. detachm	mucosa	the mouth	e	Upper jaw	Alv. c/jaw.	Total	%
Musculoskeletal	BGM	13	13	5	2	-	1	34	43,0
	Subaltern	6	3	2	1	-	-	12	15,2
	nodder	4	2	1	3	-	-	10	12,7
Cutaneous fascial	Nasolabial	5	3	-	-	-	1	9	11,4
Dermatocutaneous	Submental	-	2	1	1	-	-	4	5,1
	Cervical	3	-	-	-	-	-	3	3,8
	Dpl	1	1	-	-	-	-	2	2,5

	Frontal	-	-	-	-	2	-	2	2,5
Others	Cheek mucosa	1	2	-	-	-	-	3	3,8
Total		33 (4…	26 (3…	9 (11…	7	8	2 (2,	2 (2,	79	100

Based on the data in Table 26, it is evident that skin and muscle flaps were most frequently used for reconstruction of oral cavity defects: on the pectoralis major muscle - 34 (43.0%) cases, on the hyoid muscle - 12 (15.2%) and on the sternoclavicular-papillary muscle - 10 (12.7%) cases, which together accounted for 70.9% of the grafts used.

The proportion of skin-fascial and skin-fat flaps was 29.1%, of which the nasolabial flap was used most frequently - in 9 (11.4%) cases, submental and cervical flaps were used in almost equal frequencies - in 4 (5.1%) and 3 (3.8%) cases. The deltopectoral and frontal flaps were used less frequently, with 2 cases of each, accounting for 2.5%. Flaps from the cheek mucosa were also used in 3 (3.8%) cases to close defects of the retromolar region of the cheek.

The most frequent defects were formed in the area of the mandibular alveolar process - 33 (41.8%) cases and cheek mucosa - 26 (32.9%), less frequently in the floor of the mouth - 9 (11.4%) observations and tongue - 7 (8.9%). Defects of the maxilla and alveolar process were observed in equal frequencies in 2 (2.5%) cases each. In all cases, the reconstructive stage was included in the total duration of the surgical intervention, so the total duration of the operations, depending on the volume and type of reconstruction, ranged from 3.5 to 5.5 hours, with an average duration of 4.7 hours.

As an illustration, we present the possibilities and results of skin-muscle flap plasty on BGM:

Patient KH., born in 1939, (77 years old), pensioner, came to RONC on 20.01.2016 with complaints of a mucosal tumour of the left cheek with growth into the alveolar process of the mandible, severe pain and difficulty in opening the mouth and eating, general weakness and malaise. On examination, an ulceroinfiltrative form of exophytic tumour measuring 3.0x2.0 cm, sharply painful on palpation with irradiation to the left side of the face, which does not allow to open the mouth completely (trismus of the II degree), is detected on the mucous membrane of the left cheek with transition to the alveolar process of the mandible (Figure 34). In the left submandibular region, a dense lymph node measuring 2.0x1.0 cm with surrounding tissues of metastatic nature was palpated. A biopsy from the primary tumour was taken and fine-needle aspiration biopsy of submandibular lymph node was performed (#286 dated 20.01.2016 - Squamous cell carcinoma G1, cytogram fits into the metastasis of squamous cell carcinoma), which verified the malignant nature of the tumour. The patient was registered at RONC with the diagnosis "Cancer of the mucous membrane of the left cheek T4N1M0 stage IV (outpatient card No. 841/16)". On 25.01.2020 he was admitted to the department of general oncology (medical history №553) for further examination and development of treatment tactics. Taking into account the high degree of tumour differentiation, the patient was recommended to undergo surgical intervention at the first stage of complex treatment.

After a thorough examination by specialists of related fields, the patient was found to have a number of concomitant diseases, in particular CHD, arterial hypertension 2 degree risk 3, cholecystitis, chronic left-sided pyelonephritis, renal microlithiasis, prostatitis. To correct these disorders, the patient underwent surgical intervention (#32-34) on 02.02.2016 in the scope of Kreil's operation on the left side, excision of the left cheek mucosa tumour, marginal dissection of the lower jaw on the left side, plasty of the defect with a skin and muscle BGM flap. The total duration of the operation was 220 minutes.

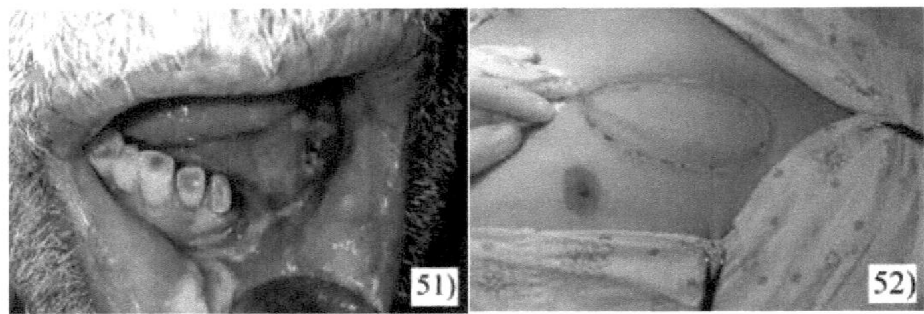

Figure 51. Left cheek mucosal tumour with extension to the mandibular alveolar process

Figure 52. Stage of the operation - marking of the skin flap site

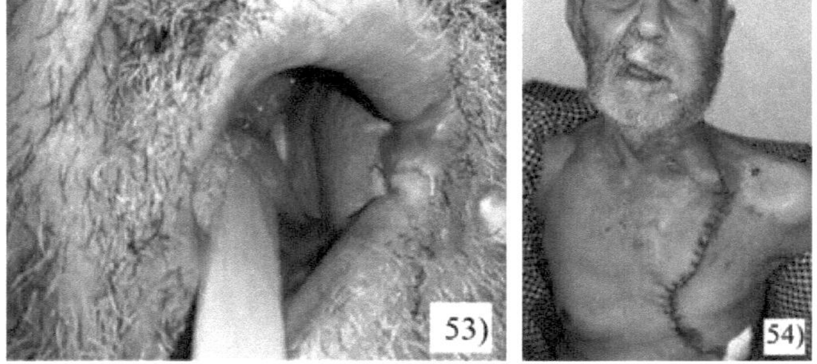

Figure 53. View of the flap on the 13th day after surgery. The cheek defect was replaced with a musculocutaneous flap on BGM

Figure 54. View of the donor site

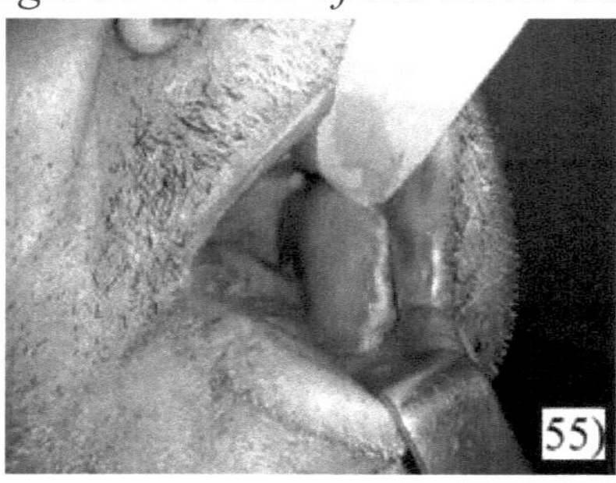

Figure 55. View of the flap 1 month after surgery

The postoperative period proceeded without peculiarities. The patient was on tube feeding. The wound healed by primary

tension with good integration of the flap on the replaced area of the cheek defect. The sutures were removed on the 9th day. Pathohistological report No. 7363 dated 06.02.2016 - squamous cell keratinising carcinoma G2 with metastases in 3 lymph nodes of the cervical fibre. The patient was discharged on 17.02.2016 on the 14th day in relatively satisfactory condition. The patient received adjuvant radiotherapy on the area of regional metastasis SOD 40 Gray and further was under dispensary observation until 09.06.2016 (date of death),
   which occurred due to cardiac disease.
of insufficiency.

4.2. Comparative characteristics of quality of life parameters of operated patients depending on the method of reconstruction

Surgical intervention for head and neck cancers in most cases causes anatomical changes that can lead to serious dysfunctions in the investigated area, such as difficulty in speech, chewing, swallowing. In addition, surgical intervention in the head and neck region also affects the appearance of the patient, causing persistent anatomo-functional and aesthetic disturbances, which are the cause of additional suffering of patients that negatively affect their quality of life. These undesirable conditions occur at different stages of combined and complex methods of treatment of patients with head and neck tumours. In the available literature there are works devoted to the problems of quality of life of patients with head and neck organ cancer. These publications fragmentarily reflect the changes in the quality of life during combined and complex treatment, which along with surgical intervention includes the effects on the patient's body of chemoradiation therapy, the side effects of which, according to many studies, have a pronounced negative impact on the patient's body.

Thus, our study was aimed at a more focused and systematic approach to investigate the effect of surgical technique on the improvement of patients' QOL parameters in locally advanced head and neck cancer, with emphasis on reconstructive and restorative techniques with arterialised pedicled flaps in different groups of patients, in order to add to the vacuum of existing studies on this problem.

Following the purpose of our study, the patients were divided into two groups - the main group, where the patients underwent tumour excision surgery with one-stage reconstruction of the defect with various arterialised flaps, and the control group, where the patients underwent only tumour excision surgery and the defect was restored by simple suturing of the wound edges or local tissue plasty. The quality of life of patients in both groups was assessed perioperatively in 2 stages - immediately before and after surgical intervention.

We studied the parameters of patients' quality of life by assessing the initial condition of patients before and after treatment. For this purpose, the general condition of patients before and after surgical intervention was determined in both groups using the Karnofskiy Performance Status Scale (0-100 points) and ECOG scale (0-4 points) (Table 27).

As shown in Table 27, the initial general condition of the patients in the main and control groups before the surgical stage of treatment were at the same level - in the range between 40 and 80 points on the Karnofsky scale.

Normal physical activity with preservation of moderately expressed symptoms of oncological disease - 80 points - took place in 23 (21.2%) patients of the main group and in 17 (27.8%) patients of the control group. At a similar level, 52 (48.2%) patients in the main group and 30 (49.1%) patients in the control group had limitations of normal activity related to the symptoms of the disease (70 points). These patients were self-maintained but were incapable of normal activity or work. In our study, the baseline condition of patients in the main and control groups were almost similar (Table 27).

Table 27. - Distribution and evaluation of the baseline status of head and neck cancer patients according to the Karnofsky index before surgery in the main and control patients

group

Characterisation of condition	Study groups		Scores	Characterisation
	Main (n=108)	Control (n = 61)		
Normal physical activity, the patient does not need special care	-	-	100	Condition is normal, no complaints or symptoms of illness
	-	-	90	Normal activity is preserved, but minor symptoms of the disease are present
	23 (21,2%)	17 (27,8%)	80	Normal activity is possible when additional efforts, with moderate symptoms of the disease
Restriction of normal activity while maintaining	52 (48,2%)	30 (49,1%)	70	The patient maintains self-care but is unable to perform normal activities or work
complete independence of the patient	24 (22,2%)	13 (21,3%)	60	The patient sometimes needs help, but is mostly self-cared for
	21 (10%)	16 (12%)	50	The patient often requires assistance and medical care
The patient is unable to care for himself/herself and requires nursing care or hospitalisation	9 (8,3%)	1 (1,6%)	40	The patient spends most of his time in bed. specialised care and assistance

Note: No statistically significant differences were found between groups using the Mann-Whitney test.

Also, 24 (22.2%) patients from the main group and 13 (21.3%) patients from the control group sometimes needed help from outsiders (60 points), and 21 (10%) patients from the main group and 16 (12%) patients from the control group often needed help and medical care - 50 points. 9 (8.3%) patients from the main group and 1 (1.6%) from the control group spent most of their time in bed, who needed extraneous help and special medical care. The significance of the difference between the preoperative Mann-Whitney U-criterion scores in both groups is shown in Table 28.

Table 28. - Results of statistical analysis of the baseline general status by the Karnofsky index in the main and control groups before <u>surgery in median quartiles Me [25q; 75q]</u>

Karnofsky index	Main group(n =108)	Control group (n =61)	P
	70,0 [60,0; 70,0]	70,0 [70,0; 80,0]	=0,1653 (>0,05; Z =-1,4)

Note: p - statistical significance of the difference between the main and control groups (by Mann-Whitney U-criterion).

This table (#28) shows that absolute values do not give significant differences between the groups *(p* = 0.1653), therefore, we analysed by qualitative parameters (in %), comparing qualitative indicators by Pearson's %2 criterion (Table 29).

Table 29. - Results of statistical analysis of the initial level of the general status of patients according to the Karnovsky index in the main and control groups <u>before surgery</u>

Karnofsky index	Main group (n = 108)	Control group (n = 61)	P
50	0,8% (9)	1,6% (1)	=0,0765 (>0,05; /' =3,1)
60	22,2% (24)	21,3% (13)	=0,8906 (>0,05; / =0,02)
70	48,2% (52)	49,2% (30)	=0,8974 (>0,05; / =0,02)
80	21,3% (23)	27,9% (17)	=0,3343 (>0,05; / =0,9)

Note: p - statistical significance of the difference between the main and control groups (by Pearson's $\%^2$ criterion).

As can be seen from Table 30, the p value > 0.05 in all comparative samples, indicating that the difference in the initial level of the general condition of patients in the main and control groups according to the Karnovsky index before surgery is statistically insignificant. The assessment of the general condition of patients after surgery according to the Karnovsky index in the main and control groups is shown in Table 30.

Table 30. - General condition of patients of the main and control groups according to the Karnovsky index after surgery

State characteristic	Study groups		Scores	Characterisation
	Main (n=108) %	Control (n = 61) %		
Normal physical activity, the patient does not need special care	6 (5,6%)	1 (1,6%)	100	Condition is normal, no complaints or symptoms of illness
	64 (59,2%)	22 (36,0%)	90	Normal activity is preserved, but minor symptoms of the disease are present
	36 (33,3%)	31 (50,8%)	80	Normal activity is possible when additional efforts, with moderate symptoms of the disease
Restriction of normal activity while maintaining the patient's complete independence	2 (1,9%)	6 (9,8%)	70	The patient is self-maintaining, but is not able to normal activities or work
	-	1 (1,63%)	60	The patient sometimes needs help, but is mostly self-sufficient

When reviewing the data in Table 30, it can be seen that after surgical intervention, the general condition of the patients in both groups generally improved by a range of 60 to 100 points. At the same time, 6 (5.6%) patients from the main group and 1

(1.6%) from the control group had their complaints and symptoms completely relieved. Minor symptoms of the disease with preserved activity were noted in 64 (59.2%) patients from the main group and 22 (36.0%) from the control group. Thirty-six (33.3%) patients from the main group and 31 (50.8%) patients from the control group retained moderately severe symptoms of the disease but were able to move with additional effort. 2 (1.9%) patients from the main group and 6 (9.8%) patients from the control group maintained self-care but were not capable of normal activities, and only 1 (1.63%) patient occasionally needed external assistance from nursing staff. The results of statistical analysis of the differences in Karnofsky index scores in both groups after surgery are shown in Table 31.

Table 31. - Significance of the difference between the indicators of both groups by Mann-Whitney U-criterion in median quartiles Me [25q; 75q]

Index	Main group (n =108)	Control group (n =61)	P
Karnofsky	90,0 [80,0; 90,0]	80,0 [80,0; 90,0]	=0,0002 (<0,001; Z =3,7)

Note: p - statistical significance of the difference between the main and control groups (by Mann-Whitney U-criterion).

As shown in Table 31, the *p* value = 0.0002, indicating statistical significance of the postoperative Karnofsky index in comparable groups. Since a qualitative analysis was performed for the preoperative values, a similar analysis was performed for the postoperative values to identify the predominance of patients (Table 32).

Table 32. - Results of statistical analysis of the general condition of patients according to the Karnovsky index after surgery (%)

Karnofsky index	Main group % (n = 108)	Control group % (n = 61)	P
60	0	1,6% (1)	-
70	1,9% (2)	9,8% (6)	=0,0189 (<0,05; /_' =5,5)
80	33,3% (36)	50,8% (31)	=0,0256 (<0,05; /2 =5,0)
90	59,3% (64)	36,1% (22)	=0,0038 (<0,01; /2 =8,4)
100	5,6% (6)	1,6% (1)	=0,2198 (>0,05; /2 =1,5)

Note: p - statistical significance of the difference between the main and control groups (by Pearson's $\%^2$ criterion).

Statistical analysis of the obtained results of the general condition of the patients after surgery revealed that statistically significant were the changes in the range from 70 to 90 points on the Karnofsky index, which was generally achieved in 102 (97.2%) patients from the main group and 59 (96.7%) patients from the control group according to Pearson's $u2$. The results of statistical analysis of the Karnofsky index scores in the main group compared before and after surgery are presented in Tables 33 and 34.

Table 33. - Results of statistical analysis of the general condition of the main group patients according to the Karnofsky index before and after the operation by median quartiles <u>Me [25q; 75q]</u>

Karnofsky index	Before surgery (n =108)	After surgery (n =108)	P
	70,0 [60,0; 70,0]	90,0 [80,0; 90,0]	$=0$,0000 (<0,001; Z =9,0)

Note: p - statistical significance of the difference between the indicators before and after surgery (Wilcoxon's T-criterion).

Table 34. - Results of statistical analysis of the general condition of the main group patients according to the Karnovsky index before and after the operation

Karnofsky index	Before surgery (n =108)	After surgery (n =108)	P
50	0,8% (9)	0	-
60	22,2% (24)	0	-
70	48,2% (52)	1,8% (2)	=0.0000 (<0.001; X^2

			=98.2)
80	21,3% (23)	33,3% (36)	=0,0008 (<0,001; /2 =11,3)
90	0	59,3% (64)	-
100	0	5,6% (6)	-

Note: p - statistical significance of the difference between the indicators before and after the operation (by the criterion of $\%^2$ McNemar).

In general, it was possible to improve the results from the range of 50 to 80 Karnofsky index scores to 70-90 scores, but the changes within the range of 70-80 scores were statistically significant. Comparative results of statistical analysis of the Karnofsky index scores in the control group before and after surgery are presented in Tables 35 and 36.

Table 35. - Results of statistical analysis of the general condition of the control group patients according to the Karnofsky index before and after surgery by the median quartiles <u>Me [25q; 75q]</u>

Index Karnofsky	Before surgery (n =61)	After surgery (n =61)	P
	70,0 [70,0; 80,0]	80,0 [80,0; 90,0]	=0,0000 (<0,001; Z =6,7]

Note: p - statistical significance of the difference between pre- and postoperative indicators (by T-criterion)
Wilcoxon).

Table 36. - Results of statistical analysis of the general condition of the control group patients according to the Karnovsky index before and after the operation

Karnofsky index	Before surgery (n =61)	After surgery (n =61)	P
50	1,6% (1)	0	
60	21,3% (13)	1,6% (1)	=0.0000 (<0.001; x^2 =55.1)
70	49,2% (30)	9,8% (6)	=0.0000 (<0.001; $\%^2$ =37.8)
80	27,9% (17)	50,8% (31)	=0,0009 (<0,001; /' =11,1)
90	0	36,1% (22)	

100	0	1,6% (1)	

Note: p - statistical significance of the difference between the indicators before and after the operation (by the criterion of $\%^2$ McNemar).

As can be seen from Tables 35 and 36, the control group also showed positive dynamics in the results in the direction of improvement - from the range of 50-80 points on the Karnofsky index to 60-100 points, but statistically significant were the changes that occurred in the range of 60-80 points.

The functional status (ECOG Status) of patients with locally advanced head and neck tumour in terms of work capacity, self-care ability, performance of daily activities and physical activity (walking, working, etc.) in the main and control groups is presented in Table 37.

Table 37. - ECOG performance status
of patients in the main and control groups before surgery

ECOG Status	Groups studied		Characterisation of condition
	Main (n =108)	Control (n =61)	
0	-	-	The patient is fully active, able to do all the things he did before the disease
1	75 (69,5%)	47 (77,0%)	The patient is unable to do heavy work, but can do light or sedentary work (e.g. light housework).
2	33 (30,5%)	14 (22,9%)	The patient is treated on an outpatient basis, is capable of self-care, but is unable to perform work. Spends more than 50% of waking time in an active upright position
3	-	-	The patient is capable of only limited self-care, spends more than 50% of waking time in a chair or bed
4	-	-	Disabled, totally incapable of self-care, bedridden.

The data in Table 37 suggest that the performance status of patients in both the main and comparison groups before surgery were almost consistent with each other on the ECOG scale. The performance status of 75 (69.5%) patients from the main group and 47 (77.0%) from the control group corresponded to an ECOG - 1 score, which correlates to a 7080 score on the Karnofsky scale and means that these patients were limited in physical strenuous activity but could perform light or sedentary office work. The work capacity of 33 (30,5%) patients from the main group and 14 (22,9%) from the control group corresponded to ECOG - 2 points, they were capable of self-care, but due to the severity of symptoms of tumour disease they could not perform work and spent more than 50% of their waking time actively in hospital. The results of statistical analysis of the ECOG status of the patients before surgery in the main and control groups are shown in Tables 38 and 39.

Table 38. - Results of statistical analysis of ECOG status indicators of patients in the studied groups before surgery by Mann-Whitney U-criterion (Me [25q; 75q])

ECOG status	Main group (n =108)	Control group (n =61)	P
	1,0 [1,0; 2,0]	1,0 [1,0; 1,0]	=0,2917 (>0,05; Z =1,0)

Note: p - statistical significance of the difference between the main and control groups (by Mann-Whitney U-criterion).

Table 39. - Results of analysis of ECOG-status indicators of patients in the studied groups before surgery by qualitative parameters (%) according to the criterion y^2.

ECOG status	Main group (n =108)	Control group (n =61)	P
0	0	0	
1	69,4% (75)	77,1% (47)	=0,2893 (>0,05; / =1,1)
2	30,6% (33)	22,9% (14)	=0,2893 (>0,05; / =1,1)
3	0	0	

Note: p - statistical significance of the difference between the main and control groups (by Pearson's y criterion[2]).

Analysing Tables 38 and 39, it can be seen that the *p* value is >

0.05, indicating statistical insignificance of differences between the studied groups before surgery in terms of ECOG status. The postoperative ECOG status of the patients in the main and control groups is summarised in Table 40.

Table 40. - ECOG performance status of patients in the main and control groups after surgery.

ECOG Status	Groups studied		Characterisation of condition
	Main (n =108) %	Control (n =61) %	
0	69 (63,8%)	23 (37,7%)	The patient is fully active, able to do all the things he did before the disease
1	39 (36,1%)	37 (60,7%)	The patient is unable to do heavy work, but can do light or sedentary work (e.g. light housework or clerical work
2	0	1 (1,6%)	The patient is treated on an outpatient basis, is capable of self-care, but is unable to perform work. More than 50% of the time awake and alert active - upright
3	-	-	The patient is capable of only limited self-care, spends more than 50% of waking time in a chair or bed
4	-	-	Disabled, totally incapable of self-care, bedridden.

After the operation, the ECOG performance status of patients in both groups changed towards improvement. At the same time, 69 (63.8%) patients from the main group and 23 (37.7%) from the control group had a better performance status.

corresponded to ECOG - 0 score, these patients were active in the postoperative period and performed everything they did before the disease. ECOG status - 1 point was returned to 39 (36.1%) patients from the main group and 37 (60.7%) from the control group. These patients could perform light sedentary work but could not take up heavy work. 1 (1.6%) patient in the control group with ECOG status - 2 points could not perform work but was capable of self-care. These results clearly demonstrate   that surgical intervention is the best way to improve the quality of life of the patient.

contributed to the improvement of patients' performance in normalised and moderate physical activity in both study groups, but this positive trend was noticeably more pronounced in the main group compared to the control group. When these results were statistically analysed, positive dynamics in the indices was also noted (Tables 41-42).

Table 41. - Results of statistical analysis of ECOG status indicators of patients in the studied groups after surgery (Me [25q; 75q])

ECOG status	Main group (n =108)	Control group (n =61)	P
	0 [0; 1,0]	1,0 [0; 1,0]	=0,0008 (<0,001; Z =-3,3)

Note: p - statistical significance of the difference between the main and control groups (by Mann-Whitney U-criterion).

Table 42. - Results of analysis of ECOG-status indicators of patients in the studied groups after surgery by qualitative parameters (%)

ECOG status	Main group (n =108)	Control group (n =61)	P
0	63,9% (69)	37,7% (23)	=0,0010 (<0,01; X^2
			=10,8)
1	36,1% (39)	60,7% (37)	=0,0021 (<0,01; /J =9,5)
2	0	1,6% (1)	
3	0	0	

Note: p - statistical significance of the difference between the main and control groups (by Pearson's $\%^2$ criterion).

As a result, we managed to change the ECOG-status of patients from low ECOG-1, 2 to ECOG-0 in 69 (63,9%) patients of the main group and 23 (37,7%) of the control group. There were 39

(36.1%) patients with relatively low ECOG-1 status in the main group and 37 (60.7%) in the control group. These differences were statistically significant (P < 0.05).

We observed that 100 (92.5%) patients from the main group and 47 (77.0%) from the control group completed the EORTC-QLQ-H&N-35 quality of life questionnaires the day before preoperative and postoperative. Clinical information was extracted from the medical records. The results of statistical analysis of the questionnaires in the main and control groups are comparatively summarised in Table 43.

Table 43. - Results of comparative statistical analysis of the results of preoperative questionnaires of patients in the main and control groups

Symptoms	Main group (n = 100)	Control group (n = 47)	*P*
Pain	41,7 [29,2; 66,7]	41,7 [25,0; 58,3]	=0,2466 (>0,05; Z =1,2)
Swallowing disorder	16,7 [8,3; 25,0]	25,0 [8,3; 33,3]	=0,0152 (<0,05; Z =-2,4)
Impaired sense of smell and taste sensitivity	16,7 [16,7; 33,3]	33,3 [16,7; 50,0]	=0,0015 (<0,01; Z =-3,3)
Speech disorder	44,4 [22,2; 44,4]	55,6 [33,3; 66,7]	=0,0008 (<0,001; Z =-3,4)
Difficulty in eating	50,0 [41,7; 66,7]	66,7 [50,0; 75,0]	=0,0023 (<0,01; Z =-3,1)
Social functioning	56,7 [46,7; 66,7]	73,3 [53,3; 80,0]	=0,0010 (<0,001; Z =-3,3)
Sexual desire	0	0	-
Dental problems	66,7 [33,3; 66,7]	66,7 [33,3; 66,7]	=0,4157 (>0,05; Z =-0,9)
Restriction of mouth opening	33,3 [33,3; 66,7]	33,3 [33,3; 33,3]	=0,0750 (>0,05; Z =1,9)
Dry mouth	33,3 [16,7; 66,7]	33,3 [33,3; 66,7]	=0,6296 (>0,05; Z =-0,5)
Saliva viscosity	33,3 [33,3; 66,7]	33,3 [33,3; 66,7]	=0,5387 (>0,05; Z =0,7)
Coughing	0	0 [0; 33,3]	-
Feeling sick	66,7 [66,7;	100,0 [66,7;	=0,0052 (<0,01; Z

	100,0]	100,0]	=-3,1)
Pain management	0	0	
Food additives	100,0 [100,0;100,0]	100,0 [0; 100,0]	=0,0373 (<0,05; Z =3,0)
Nasogastric tube	100,0 [100,0;100,0]	0 [0; 100,0]	=0,0000 (<0,001; Z =8,3
Loss of the cape	0	0	
Weight increase	100,0 [100,0; 00,0]	100,0 [100,0;100,0]	=0,9127 (>0,05; Z =0,5)

Note: p - statistical significance of the difference between the main and control groups (by Mann-Whitney U-criterion). (Me [25q; 75q])

Thus, it follows from this table that before surgery, the patients in both groups did not differ significantly in terms of the level of impairment of the QOL parameters. Of these, the severity of pain, use of analgesics, problem chewing hard food, missing teeth, trismus of the masticatory muscles, feeling of dry mouth and viscosity of saliva, and weight loss were at the same level in patients of both groups before surgery. Despite this, the questionnaire revealed some statistically significant differences in the intensity of one or another symptom more pronounced in the

control group. Thus, difficulties with the act of swallowing, sense of smell, speaking, eating in the community, social contact and general feeling of illness prevailed in patients of the control group. Comparative analyses of postoperative questionnaire results in both groups are summarised in median quartiles in Table 44.

Table44 . - Results of comparative statistical analysis of the results of postoperative questionnaires of patients in the main and control groups (Me [25q; 75q])

Symptoms	Main group (n =100)	Control group (n =47)	P
Pain	8,3 [8,3; 16,7]	33,3 [25,0; 50,0]	=0,0000 (<0,001; Z =-7,6)
Swallowing disorder	8,3 [0; 8,3]	25,0 [8,3;	=0,0000 (<0,001;

		33,3]	Z =-6,1)
Impaired sense of smell and taste sensitivity	16,7 [0; 3,3]	33,3 [16,7; 50,0]	=0,0000 (<0,001; Z =-4,8)
Speech disorder	22,2 [11,1; 22,2]	55,6 [33,3; 66,7]	=0,0000 (<0,001; Z =-7,2)
Difficulty in eating	25,0 [25,0; 33,3]	66,7 [50,0; 75,0]	=0,0000 (<0,001; Z =-7,5)
Social functioning	26,7 [20,0; 33,3]	73,3 [53,3; 80,0]	=0,0000 (<0,001; Z =-7,9)
Sexual desire	0	0	
Dental problems	66,7 [33,3; 66,7]	66,7 [33,3; 66,7]	=0,0533 (>0,05; Z =-2,1)
Restriction of mouth opening	33,3 [0; 33,3]	33,3 [33,3; 33,3]	=0,0012 (<0,01; Z =-3,6)
Dry mouth	0 [0; 33,3]	33,3 [33,3; 66,7]	=0,0000 (<0,001; Z =-6,8)
Saliva viscosity	0 [0; 33,3]	33,3 [33,3; 66,7]	=0,0000 (<0,001; Z =-5,8)
Coughing	0 [0; 33,3]	0 [0; 33,3]	=0,1007 (>0,05; Z =-2,0)
Feeling sick	33,3 [33,3; 33,3]	100,0 [66,7; 100,0]	=0,0000 (<0,001; Z =-8,3)
Pain management	100,0 [100,0; 100,0]	0	
Food additives	100,0 [0; 100,0]	100,0 [0; 100,0]	=0,8143 (>0,05; Z =0,3)
Nasogastric tube	0 [0; 100,0]	0 [0; 100,0]	=0,7492 (>0,05; Z =-0,4)
Weight loss	0 [0; 100,0]	0	
Weight gain	100,0 [100,0; 100,0]	100.0 (unchanged)	

Note: p - statistical significance of the difference between the main and control groups (by Mann-Whitney U-criterion).

This analysis shows that there were statistically significant changes in pain intensity, impaired swallowing, smell and taste, free mouth opening, xerostomia, salivary viscosity, speech, eating in public places, social contact, and feeling of general soreness between the patient groups after surgery.

Having studied in detail these changes within the study groups, it can be seen that, in general, we were able to make positive adjustments in almost all the parameters of the QOL of the patients in the main group (Table 45).

Table 45. - Statistical analysis of the questionnaire results of the main group patients before and after surgery (Me [25q; 75q])

Symptoms	Before surgery (n =100)	After surgery (n =99)	P
Pain	41,7 [29,2; 66,7]	8,3 [8,3; 16,7]	=0,0000 (<0,001; Z =8,0)
Swallowing disorder	16,7 [8,3; 25,0]	8,3 [0; 8,3]	=0,0000 (<0,001; Z =5,2)
Impaired sense of smell and taste sensitivity	16,7 [16,7; 33,3]	16,7 [0; 3,3]	=0,0044 (<0,01; Z =2,8)
Speech disorder	44,4 [22,2; 44,4]	22,2 [11,1; 22,2]	=0,0000 (<0,001; Z =6,9)
Difficulty in eating	50,0 [41,7; 66,7]	25,0 [25,0; 33,3]	=0,0000 (<0,001; Z =7,7)
Social functioning	56,7 [46,7; 66,7]	26,7 [20,0; 33,3]	=0,0000 (<0,001; Z =8,0)
Sexual desire	0	0	
Dental problems	66,7 [33,3; 66,7]	66,7 [33,3; 66,7]	=0,7222 (>0,05; Z =0,4)
Restriction of mouth opening	33,3 [33,3; 66,7]	33,3 [0; 33,3]	=0,0000 (<0,001; Z =5,8)
Dry mouth	33,3 [16,7; 66,7]	0 [0; 33,3]	=0,0000 (<0,001; Z =6,5)
Saliva viscosity	33,3 [33,3; 66,7]	0 [0; 33,3]	=0,0000 (<0,001; Z =6,6)
Coughing	0	0 [0; 33,3]	
Feeling sick	66,7 [66,7; 100,0]	33,3 [33,3; 33,3]	=0,0000 (<0,001; Z =7,5)
Pain management	0	100,0 [100,0;100,0]	-
Food additives	100,0 [100,0; 100,0]	100,0 [0; 100,0]	=0,0021 (<0,01; Z =3,1)
Nasogastric tube	100,0 [100,0; 100,0]	0 [0; 100,0]	=0,0000 (<0,001; Z =7,2)
Weight loss	0	0 [0; 100,0]	
Weight gain	100,0 [100,0; 100,0]	100,0 [100,0; 100,0]	=0,1088 (>0,05; Z =1,6)

Note: p - statistical significance of the difference between the indicators before and after surgery (Wilcoxon's T-criterion).

All patients in the main group reported statistically significant positive changes in the degree of severity of symptoms of the disease. Dental problems and changes in body weight remained unchanged, which should be taken into account in further management of patients of this contingent. We also analysed the results of the questionnaire in the control group before and after surgery (Table 46).

Table 46. - Statistical analysis of questionnaire results of control group patients before and after surgery (Me [25q; 75q])

Symptom	Before surgery (n =47)	After surgery (n =46)	P
Pain	41,7 [25,0; 58,3]	33,3 [25,0; 50,0]	=0,6891 (>0,05; Z =0,4)
Swallowing disorder	25,0 [8,3; 33,3]	25,0 [8,3; 33,3]	=0,2604 (>0,05; Z =1,1)
Impaired sense of smell and taste sensitivity	33,3 [16,7; 50,0]	33,3 [16,7; 50,0]	=0,8886 (>0,05; Z =0,1)
Speech disorder	55,6 [33,3; 66,7]	55,6 [33,3; 66,7]	=0,7299 (>0,05; Z =0,3)
Difficulty in eating	66,7 [50,0; 75,0]	66,7 [50,0; 75,0]	=0,9750 (>0,05; Z =0,0)
Social functioning	73,3 [53,3; 80,0]	73,3 [53,3; 80,0]	=0,5563 (>0,05; Z =0,6)
Sexual desire	0	0	
Dental problems	66,7 [33,3; 66,7]	66,7 [33,3; 66,7]	=0,5286 (>0,05; Z =0,6)
Restriction of mouth opening	33,3 [33,3; 33,3]	33,3 [33,3; 33,3]	=0,5002 (>0,05; Z =0,7)
Dry mouth	33,3 [33,3; 66,7]	33,3 [33,3; 66,7]	=0,7531 (>0,05; Z =0,3)
Saliva viscosity	33,3 [33,3; 66,7]	33,3 [33,3; 66,7]	=0,5337 (>0,05; Z =0,6)
Coughing	0 [0; 33,3]	0 [0; 33,3]	=0,5286 (>0,05; Z =0,6)
Feeling sick	100,0 [66,7; 100,0]	100,0 [66,7; 100,0]	=0,7989 (>0,05; Z =0,2)
Pain management	0	0	
Food additives	100,0 [0; 100,0]	100,0 [0; 100,0]	=1,0000 (>0,05; Z

			=0)
Nasogastric tube	0 [0; 100,0]	0 [0; 100,0]	=0,3454 (>0,05; <u>Z</u> <u>=0,9)</u>
Weight loss	0	0	-
Weight gain	100,0 [100,0; 100,0]	100.0 (no variance)	-

Note: p - statistical significance of the difference between the indicators before and after surgery (Wilcoxon's T-criterion).

Thus, the quality of life measured by the EORTC QLQ-H&N-35 questionnaire showed no significant differences between the different patient groups preoperatively. However, postoperatively, overall, patients in the main group who underwent reconstruction using arterialised pedicle flaps reported a better quality of life compared to the control group. In addition, the results showed that patients in the 2 groups had relatively high scores on physical functioning, role functioning, and global quality of life, whereas they scored lower on emotional and cognitive functioning. Among symptoms, the most bothersome symptoms in the main group were pain, chewing associated with missing teeth, while in the control group, pain, senses of smell and taste, missing teeth, problems in social contact in the community, and a general sense of soreness were the most bothersome symptoms.

4.3. Immediate functional and aesthetic results and survival analyses of patients

It should be noted that the incidence of postoperative complications in locally advanced head and neck cancer as a result of combined and complex treatment remains high from 70-95%. There are a number of factors contributing to the occurrence of postoperative complications. The incidence of postoperative complications directly depends on the volume of the performed operation, which in typical operations is up to 20%, and in extended combined variants reaches up to 75%.

An important factor contributing to the occurrence of

postoperative complications is the duration of surgical intervention time, the average value of which differs in the studied groups. We calculated the duration of surgery time in the compared groups and statistical analysis of the results is shown in Figure 56.

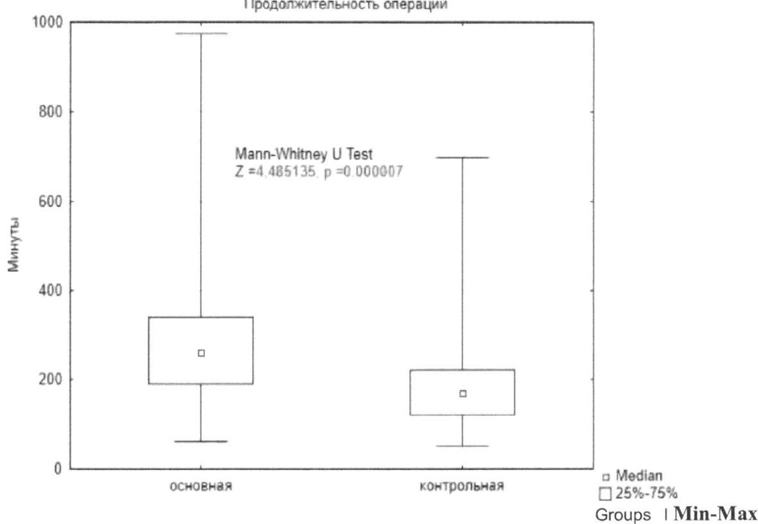

Figure 56. Duration of surgery in main and control groups in minutes (p < 0.001 by Mann-Whitney U-criterion) (Me [25q; 75q])

As can be seen from Figure 56, in the main group, the average operation lasted from 190 to 340 minutes, while in the control group from 120 to 230 minutes. This is explained by the fact that in the main group, along with the stage of tumour resection and surgery on the pathways of regional metastasis, the stage of one-stage flap reconstruction was also performed.

Postoperative complications and measures to prevent them play a significant role in assessing the results of reconstructive and reconstructive surgeries. There are general and local postoperative complications. To general complications, we considered non-specific complications associated with exhaustion of functional reserves and decreased reactivity of the patient's organism - anaemia, nutritional deficiency, weight loss up to cachexia, exacerbation of chronic concomitant disease.

Local - specific complications related to the postoperative wound and flap directly depend on the regenerative abilities and state of tissues of the patients' organism, and previously received treatment methods. All these complications are clinically significant for patients and can adversely affect the results of treatment of patients and their quality of life. Therefore, the development of measures for the prevention of the listed complications arising after surgeries of locally advanced head and neck cancer requires the study of the factors contributing to their occurrence. In our work, complications were noted in both groups and directly correlated with the tumour process stage (Table 47).

Table 47. - Frequency of postoperative complications in the studied groups depending on the stages of the disease

Reported complications	Disease stage		Total n, (%)	P
	III	**IV**		
Main group (n = 108)	13 (12,0%)	28 (25,9%)	41 (37,9%) $p=0,010$ (/2=6,774)	0.647 (/2 =0,210)
Control group (n = 61)	4 (6,5%)	17 (27,9%)	21 (34,4%) $p=0,005$ (/2=9,721)	
	$p=0.384$ (/2=0,759)	0.784 (/2=0,075)		

Note: p - statistical significance of the difference between the indicators of the main and control groups (by Pearson's $\%^2$ criterion).

The data in Table 47 show that in both groups of patients studied, complications were mainly correlated with the severity of the tumour process and were more prevalent in stage IV than in stage III, being 25.9% versus 12.0% in the main group (two-fold increase), and 27.9% versus 6.5% (4-fold increase) in the control group.

Table 48. - Distribution of patients by the nature and frequency of specific complications in the studied <u>groups</u>

Nature of local complications		Main group n = 108, (%)	Control group n = 61, (%)	P
Seam separation		-	19 (31,1%)	-
Flap necrosis	regional	6 (5,5%)	2 (3,3%)	0,771
	partial	24 (22,2%)	-	<0,001
	complete	11 (10,2%)	-	-
Total		41 (37,9%)	21 (34,4%)	0,647

Note: p - statistical significance of the difference between the indicators of the main and control groups (by Pearson's $\%^2$ criterion).

When analysing the results of treatment (Table 48), attention was drawn to the relatively high number of local complications that can affect the postoperative course of the disease and rehabilitation of patients with locally advanced head and neck cancer.

1. Wound suppuration and suture divergence in the flap and/or donor area are usually associated, first of all, with the contamination of the area around the tumour lesion, general oncological and nutritional status, and may also be a consequence of violation of aseptic principles during the stage of flap harvesting and stitching of the separated wound edges. According to the Dutch authors, the frequency of postoperative complications ranges from 22% in normally nourished patients to 56% in patients with reduced body mass index. This has the consequence of prolonging the hospitalisation time of patients.

In our study, the frequency of such complications was observed in 31.1% of cases in the control group. It should be noted that the relatively high frequency of this type of complications in the control group is most likely due to the tension of the wound edges as a consequence of a large diastasis of the edges of the defect formed.

2. The formation of orostomas and sluggish fistulas is a fairly common phenomenon in oral surgery, which is caused by the action of saliva and oral microflora. A total of 11.2% were observed in the total cohort, of which 9 (8.3%) cases were observed in the main group, and with almost double frequency in 10 (16.4%) cases in the control group.

3. Marginal and/or partial flap necrosis, i.e. loss of graft viability affecting the distal ends of the flaps in the form of necrosis of the marginal areas of the skin pad, not more than 60%. In our study the complication in the form of marginal necrosis of the flap was noted in 5.5% of the patients of the main group and 3.3% of the control group, 7 (6.5%) of the main group and 2 (3.3%) patients of the control group. Partial flap necrosis was noted in 24 (22.2%) patients of the main group. These patients underwent conservative measures to prevent further development of necrosis.

4. Complete flap necrosis - total **necrosis** of more than 60% of all layers of the working part of the flap (skin, subcutaneous tissue, fascia, muscle) involved in replenishing the formed postoperative defect. A formidable complication of this category was observed in 11 (10.2%) cases in the patients of the main group. In these cases, in order to prevent the development of further purulent-infectious complications, we performed necrectomy, which in most cases was performed from the fourth to the seventh day after surgery.

5. Bleeding, haematoma in the flap area are both early and late postoperative complications. Early bleeding occurs as a result of insufficient wound haemostasis during surgery, as well as due to slippage of the ligated vessel. Late haemorrhage is a consequence of post-radiation changes of head and neck tissues, purulent-necrotic changes and arrosion of the main vessels. Such complications occurred in 2 (1.2%) cases - 1 case in each group (0.9% and 1.6%), respectively, which caused repeated surgical interventions.

Along with specific complications, general complications were also noted: exacerbation of chronic concomitant disease was noted in 5 (4.6%) cases in the main group and 5 (8.2%) in the control group. The frequency of complications depending on the method of treatment is shown in Table 49.

Table 49. - Frequency of postoperative complications depending on the treatment tactics (n = 169)

Treatment tactics	Core group	Control group	P	Total	P(%)
hlt + Operation	12	8	0,890	20 (32,2%)	42 (24,9%)
LT + Surgery	8	7	0,541	15 (24,2%)	
XT + Surgery	7	-	-	7 (11,3%)	
Surgery + LT	5	4	0,858	9 (14,5%)	20 (11,8%)
Surgery + XT	4	1	0,774	5 (8,1%)	
Operation	5	1	0,565	6 (9,7%)	
Total	41	21	0,647	62 (100%)	62 (36,7%)
P					= 0,002 (χ^2=9,59)

Note: p - statistical significance of the difference between the indicators of the main and control groups (by Pearson's $\%^2$ criterion).

Studies have proven a directly proportional dependence of the incidence of postoperative complications on previously performed neoadjuvant chemoradiation treatment. This is explained by the fact that the effect of ionising radiation negatively affects microcirculation and regenerative-restorative processes in the tissues around the tumour. The data of Table 49 clearly show that among the patients of the main and control groups who received preoperative radiotherapy and/or chemoradiotherapy at the first stage, complications were noted twice as often (67.7% vs. 32.2%) as in patients who underwent surgery at the first stage, which dictates the necessity of transferring the surgical stage of treatment before chemoradiotherapy. We also performed a comparative analysis of the incidence of postoperative purulinonecrotic complications in the main group (n=108) of patients divided according to the time principle in retrospective and prospective subgroups (Table 50).

Table 50. - Frequency of postoperative complications in retrospective and prospective subgroup of patients in the main group (n=108)

Study groups	Retrospective group (n = 44)	Prospective group (n = 64)	Total
Specific complications	21 (47,7%)	20 (31,2%)	41
	$p = 0.083$ ($x^2 = 3.006$)		(100%)

Note: p - statistical significance of the difference between the indicators of the main and control groups (by Pearson's $\%^2$ criterion).

Complications of reconstructive-reconstructive surgery surgeries were analysed on the model of the main group (n=108) of patients, of which 64 (59.3%) were 204
were treated prospectively, and 44 (40.7%) - retrospectively. The incidence of purulent-necrotic complications in the prospective subgroup was 20 (31.2%), and in the retrospective subgroup - 21 (47.7%). The obtained results show that we managed to reduce postoperative complications by 16.5%. This indicates that the measures taken to prevent purulent-necrotic complications at all stages of surgical treatment were effective.

4.3.1 Functional and aesthetic outcomes

To assess the functional and aesthetic results of treatment, we used a 4-point scale (in the form of a questionnaire) filled out by patients after surgery, which was developed collegially by the staff of the Department of General Oncology of the State University of the Russian Oncological Centre and is used in our institution (Table 51).

Table 51. - Scale for evaluating aesthetic results

Aesthetic defect	Patient self-esteem	Scores

Slightly pronounced	Not impaired, uncomfortable interacting with strangers	4
Visible defect, scar, facial asymmetry, can be completely hidden by clothing	Reduced slightly, defect can be masked by hairstyle, glasses, clothing, limits communication	3
A noticeable defect, scarring, asymmetry, impossible to hide with clothes. Masked with a bandage	Reduced, wearing concealer in the street and at home, avoiding contact with strangers	2
Significant defect, asymmetry, cannot be completely concealed with a bandage	Disturbed, constant wearing of a masking bandage , tries not to leave the house	1

The data obtained by the questionnaire allow us to take into account the presence of pain after surgery, free opening of the mouth, chewing, swallowing, speech, ability to return to previous work, as well as the patient's overall subjective assessment of the result of surgery (Tables 52, 53).

Table 52. - Perception of the results of the operation

Perception of the results of the operation	Scores	Main group n = 108 (%)	Control group n = 61 (%)	P
It's good	4	35 (32,4)	2 (3,3)	<0.001
Satisfactory	3	40 (37,0)	8 (13,1)	0.002
Relatively satisfactory	2	27 (25,0)	43 (70,5)	<0,001
Unsatisfactory	1	4 (3,7)	8 (13,1)	0.049

Note: p - statistical significance of the difference between the indicators of the main and control groups (by Pearson's $\%^2$ criterion).

Good and satisfactory functional results were noted in 69.4% of patients in the main group and in 16.6% in the control group.

Table 53. - Aesthetic results

Evaluation of aesthetic results	Scores	Main group n = 108 (%)	Control group n = 61 (%)	P
It's good	4	20 (18,5)	2 (3,3)	0.010
Satisfactory	3	50 (46,3)	7 (11,5)	<0,001
Relatively satisfactory	2	31 (28,7)	41 (67,2)	<0,001
Unsatisfactory	1	7 (6,5)	11 (18,0)	0.038

Note: p - statistical significance of the difference between the indicators of the main and control groups (by Pearson's $\%^2$ criterion).

In aesthetic terms, good and satisfactory results were achieved in the main group in 64.8% of patients and in the control group in 14.8%.

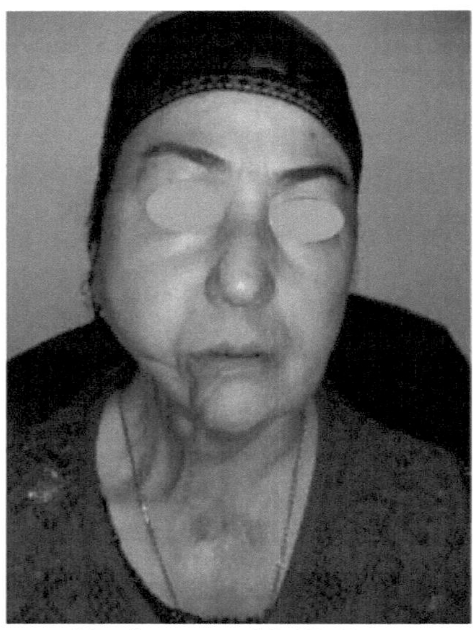

Figure 57. - Patient N., born in 1965. Diagnosis: Cancer of the mucous membrane of the alveolar process of the mandible on the right side T4N0M0IV stage. Status after surgery (September 2012).

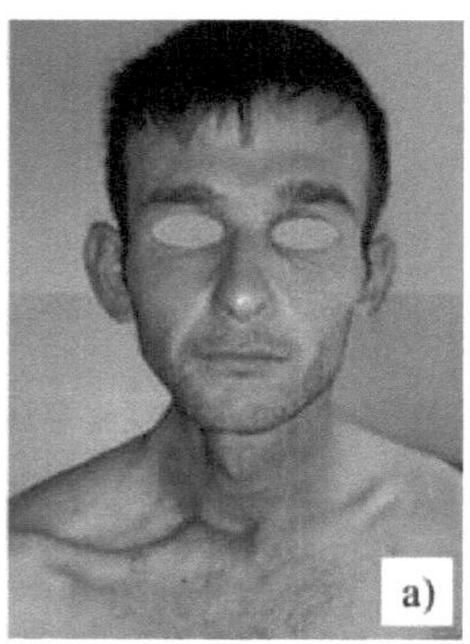

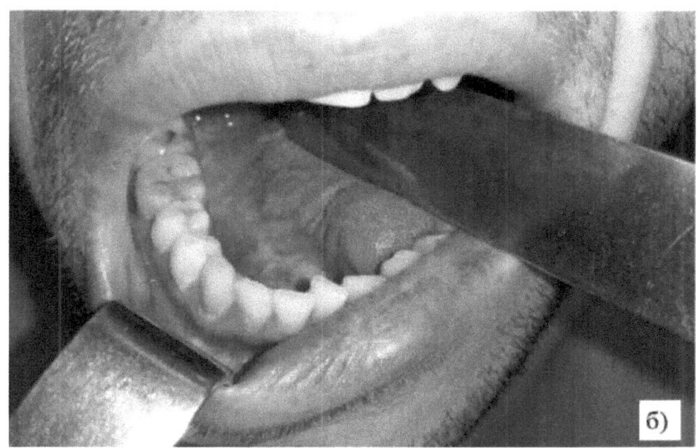

Figure 58. a) - Patient Sh., 33 years old, diagnosis: Right lateral tongue cancer T3N1M0, status after 2 courses of PCT and surgery - Tracheostomy. FFIKSH on the right side. Hemiglosectomy on the right side. Plasty of the defect with a complex musculoskeletal flap on the cieatellar muscle. (February 2012) b) local status without signs of recurrence

To calculate the overall observed survival rates, we followed the fate of all patients included in the study group by active and passive follow-up. Active follow-up included data from telephone follow-up examinations and dispensary examinations. Passive follow-up was based on data from testimonies of close relatives and death certificates of registered patients.

The starting point was the date of verification of the patients' diagnosis, and the ending point was the data on death with specification of its cause. When analysing the latter, we also included deaths not related to the tumour process, i.e. severe intercurrent (concomitant) cardiovascular pathology, which contributed to shortening the patients' lives and became 208

The reasons for obtaining did not affect the decrease in the rates of long-term results. Despite this, our data are quite comparable with the literature data. The overall observed survival in the main and control group of patients was measured at 1, 3 and 5 and 10-year intervals. The Kaplan-Meier survival plot clearly demonstrates that the overall observed survival and life expectancy of patients in the main group was significantly higher than in the control group, the magnitude of which was statistically significant (Figure 59).

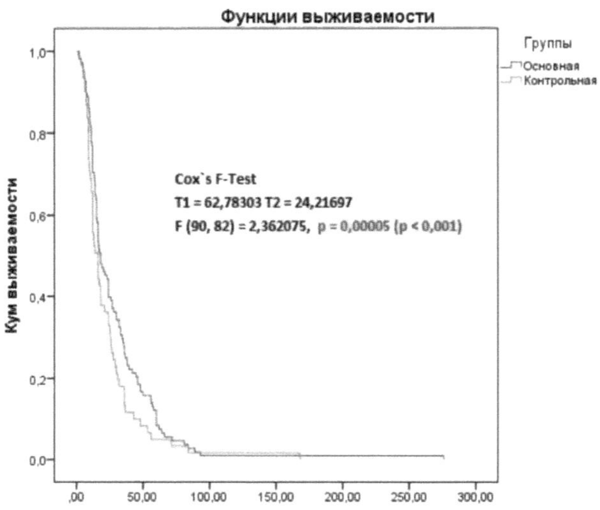

Time (months)

Figure 59. - Kaplan-Meier survival rate of the main and control group patients (p<0.001 by Cox's F-criterion)

Thus, one-year observed survival in the main and control groups was (96.1% vs. 79.9%), three-year survival was 62.2% vs. 33.7%, and 5-year survival was 33.5% vs. 13.3% (Table 54).

Table 54. - Overall observed 1-, 3-, and 5-year survival of patients in the main and control groups

Survival of patients	Main group %, (n)	Control group %, (n)	P
1-year	96,1% (89)	79,9% (49)	0,738
3-year-old	62,2% (58)	33,7% (21)	0,016
5 year old	35,5% (33)	13,3% (8)	0,019

Note: p - statistical significance of the difference between the indicators of the main and control groups (by Pearson's $\%^2$ criterion).

Table 55. - Mean and median survival times of patients in the main and control groups

groups	Average			Median		
	Time, months.	95% confidence interval		Time, months.	95% confidence interval	
		Lower boundary	Upper boundary		Lower boundary	Upper boundary
Basic	29,2	23,255	35,238	18,0	12,776	23,224
Control	22,9	16,689	29,223	16,0	11,655	20,345
Total	26,9	22,517	31,435	16,5	14,623	18,377

As can be seen from Tables 54 and 55, there is a significant difference in survival rates in the main and control groups. Our clinical observations and literature data have established that recurrences and metastases of head and neck cancer mostly occur in the first year after surgery, which is a poor prognostic factor. Consequently, the survival rate of patients in the main group after 1 year to 3 years decreased from 96.1% to 62.2% (a difference of 33.9%.), and in the control group, this rate ranged from 79.9% to 33.7% (a difference of 46.2%.). Five-year survival rate in the main group was 35.5%, and in the control group - 13.3%, which is 2.7 times less than the main group. The above data allow to judge about poor survival rate of the control group patients, which is probably caused by refusal (abstention) from reconstructive-restorative stage of surgical treatment, economical non-radical or conditionally-radical (R1 and R+) resections and as a consequence high frequency of recurrence and metastasis of tumours.

Multivariate analysis of the relationship between survival, localisation, tumour stage and defect category is shown in Tables 56-58.

Table 56. - Effect of tumour localisation on survival (n =169)

Localisation	Odds ratio (OR)	95% confidence interval		P	Note
		lower	upper		
Larynx	-	-	-	-	2 patients
Thyroid.	-	-	-	-	1 patient
Skin coverings	0,977	0,459	2,081	=0,953 (B =-0,023)	U > G
Guba	0,514	0,177	1,493	=0,221 (B =-0,665)	U < G
Upper jaw	9,143	1,167	71,658	=0,035 (B =2,213)	U > G
AHF	1,260	0,224	7,082	=0,793 (B =0,231)	U > G
Cheek	2,198	0,828	5,834	=0,114 (B =0,788)	U > G
Language	0,640	0,264	1,551	=0,232 (B =-0,446)	U > G
AHNCH	0,729	0,346	1,537	=0,407 (B =-0,316)	U > g
DPR	1,101	0,309	3,917	=0,882 (B =0,096)	U > g

Note: OR - odds ratio; AOVCH - alveolar process of the maxilla; AONCH - alveolar process of the mandible; DPR - floor of the oral cavity; U - deceased, L - survivors. p - statistical significance of the difference between the indicators of the main and control groups (by Pearson's $\%^2$ criterion).

Tumour localisation in the maxilla had a negative impact on patient survival (OR = 9.143, CI 1.16771.658, p=0.035). Other localisations - skin, lip tumours, alveolar process of the upper and lower jaw, cheek, tongue and floor of the oral cavity did not affect the survival rate of patients (p>0.05).

An analysis of the effect of tumour stage on survival is shown in Table 57.

Table 57. - Probability of influence of disease stage on survival rate

Tumour stage	Odds ratio (OR)	95% confidence interval		P	Note
		lower	upper		
II	0,354	0,130	0,967	=0,043 (B =-	U < G

				1,038)	
III	1,176	0,600	2,306	=0,637 (B =0,162)	U > g
IV	1,317	0,704	2,646	=0,389 (B =0,275)	U > g

Note: D - dead, L - survivors; OR - odds ratio. *p* - statistical significance of the difference between the indicators of the main and control groups (by Pearson's $\%^2$ criterion).

There was a positive correlation between stage II disease and survival (OR = 0, 354, CI 0.130-0.967, p=0.043). Other stages (III-IV) showed a high risk of decreased survival, with statistically insignificant p value (p=0.637, p=0.389).

Table 58. - Probability of defect category influence on survival (n=169)

Category of defects	Odds ratio (OR)	95% confidence interval		*p*	outcome
		lower	upper		
I	0,977	0,459	2,081	=0,953 (B =-0,023)	U > G
II	1,074	0,552	2,090	=0,834 (B =0,071)	U > g
III	1,622	0,487	5,405	=0,431 (B =0,484)	U > g
IV	-	-	-	-	3 patients in total

Note: D - dead, L - survivors; OR - odds ratio. *p* - statistical significance of the difference between the indicators of the main and control groups (by Pearson's $\%^2$ criterion).

There were also no statistically significant results for the effect of postoperative defect category on patient survival (p > 0.05) (Table 58).

Squamous cell cancer is about 90-95%, occupying the 6th place among malignant tumours of head and neck organs or 7% in the general morbidity structure of human malignant neoplasms and is among the ten most frequently occurring forms.

It most often develops from the epithelium of the skin and mucous membranes (oral cavity, sinuses, naso-oropharynx and larynx). Depending on the localisation, it has a diverse clinical course, which in most cases is difficult to treat and is characterised by high mortality and disability rates. The number of new cases detected for the first time every year is also increasing, of which up to 65-75% are locally advanced, i. e., locally disseminated forms.

advanced stages. In these cases, the optimal treatment tactics are combined and complex methods, among which surgical intervention has a special place. Despite the multimodality of treatment, the incidence of locoregional recurrence of head and neck squamous cell carcinoma remains high, which puzzles the use of new combinations of antitumour, targeting drugs and immunotherapeutic agents [21, 22, 31,57].

Despite all the advances in the treatment of head and neck cancers, there are a number of problems that require improvement and refinement. One of these problems is the formation of extensive postoperative defects affecting the vital body functions of patients like speech, chewing, swallowing breathing as well as decontaminating appearance and aesthetics, which is in most cases the reason for patients' rejection of the proposed treatment method [24]. Hence, 214

The main requirements for reconstructive surgery in patients with head and neck cancer are the need for one-stage closure of extensive defects with maximum restoration of anatomical integrity and functions of the lost organs and tissues. The expected ultimate goal of reconstructive interventions is not only the successful replacement of the formed defects, but also the achievement of maximum medical, psycho-emotional and social rehabilitation of the individual.

Currently, there are various methods of reconstructive interventions, which are periodically supplemented with new methods. The variety of known reconstruction techniques, individual characteristics and preferences of cancer patients, in many cases, creating new dilemmas, complicate the choice of the most optimal method of reconstruction by the surgeon. In some cases, these factors serve as a reason for not performing the reconstructive stage.

With the development and introduction into clinical practice of methods of reconstructive surgery with complex vascularised flaps on a pedicle, the indications for surgical treatment of locally advanced forms of cancer of the study area have significantly expanded. These flaps have a number of advantages:

1. Lack of concern of the oncological surgeon related to the need for defect replacement, allowing radical surgery.

2. Defects are repaired simultaneously with excision of the head and neck tumour, which significantly reduces the treatment time of patients.

3. The grafting rate of these flaps is high and is 9098%.

4. Unlike free skin flaps, they can be used in the reconstruction of wounds with non-ideal conditions, uneven surfaces of the recipient bed, exposed bone, cartilage and tendon.

5. The rich vascularisation of the flaps minimises the risk of wound infection, and in the case of the latter, flap survival is not reduced by antibiotic treatment.

6. A higher cosmetic appearance can be achieved, which is essential to improve the quality of life of patients.

7. Finally, this technique is relatively simple and does not require special expensive equipment and tools.

Despite their advantages, flaps with axial circulation have a number of disadvantages. Thus, extensive surgical resection in the area of the donor site required for mobilisation of the flap stem, the need for additional skin excision along the edge of the donor bed for additional mobilisation, as well as the use of various unloading sutures are limiting factors. Aesthetic and cosmetic features: the difference between the recipient area and the surrounding tissues (direction of hair growth, colour and length of hair coat, presence of glandular tissue or thickness of fatty tissue) are factors limiting their use.

However, new knowledge is constantly being added to this field and more frequent reports on the development and application of new flaps are appearing. It is extremely important to choose the optimal flap and method of defect reconstruction for each specific patient, which would allow to achieve maximum functional and aesthetic results and improve the quality of life. At the same time, rehabilitation after ablative surgery is an important issue that needs to be addressed.

Having analysed the available literature data, we came to the conclusion that one-stage reconstructive and restorative surgeries are an obligatory and priority component of combined and complex treatment of patients with head and neck cancer. Our work proved the effectiveness and expediency of one-stage reconstructive surgical interventions simultaneously after removal of the primary malignant tumour and on the pathways of regional metastasis.

The aim of our work was to improve the functional and cosmetic results of reconstructive and reconstructive surgeries for defects of the head and neck region after cancer surgery.

In order to achieve our goal, we have defined the following

objectives:

1. To analyse the frequency of localisations, nature and methods of reconstruction of defects after removal of head and neck organ cancers.

2. Development of an algorithm for choosing the optimal method of plasty depending on the anatomo-topographical characteristics of the flaps, localisation and category of defects.

3. To analyse the incidence of postoperative complications of reconstructive-restorative surgeries with the use of leg flaps and to develop measures for their prevention.

4. To evaluate the immediate results of defect plasty and determine their impact on the quality of life and survival of patients.

Our work is based on clinical observations of 169 patients with locally advanced head and neck cancer treated at the Republican Cancer Research Centre from 2008 to 2019. Of these, 152 patients (89.9%) had locally advanced tumour process and corresponded to stages III-IV. Men significantly prevailed over women - 107 (63.3%), against 62 (36.7%).

All patients were divided into 2 groups: main (n=108) and control (n=61), which did not differ in sex, age, stage, severity of symptoms of oncological process, concomitant diseases, socio-economic and performance status, as well as quality of life level.

The main and control groups were comparable according to the main criteria: age of patients, sex, localisation and stage of tumour process. The peak of morbidity in both groups was observed in the age categories from 45-74 years, i.e. middle-aged and elderly people prevailed. Of the concomitant diseases, the most frequent in the studied groups were pathology of the gastrointestinal tract, respectively (76.8% vs. 77.0%), inflammatory diseases of the kidneys and urinary tract (65.7%

and 59.0%), cardiovascular system (50,0% and 39.3%), anaemia of varying severity (31.4% and 34.4%), reproductive system (15.7% and 27.8%), endocrine system (13.8% and 5.0%), and various infectious and allergic diseases (viral hepatitis B, C, polyvalent allergy) 11.1% and 8.2%. We consider the age of patients and their initial somatic status to be one of the important factors in decision-making and development of treatment tactics for patients in this cohort.

All patients underwent combined and complex treatment. The analysis of the methods of reconstruction of defects after removal of squamous cell carcinoma of the head and neck organs showed that in both groups after removal of the malignant tumour there were defects of various complexity categories that required one-stage reconstruction. The main difference between the groups of patients was in the volume of the performed reconstructive intervention and the graft used to replace the defects. For this purpose in the main group (n = 108) arterialised skin-fat, skin-fascial (n = 65) and skin-muscular (n = 56) flaps on a pedicle were used. In the comparison group (n = 61) patients the restoration of the formed defects was achieved by simple suturing of the dissected wound edges, without using the above mentioned flaps, or by free skin grafts.

The most frequent sites of cancer were: the skin of the head and neck 21.3%, the alveolar process of the mandible 21.3%, the cheek mucosa 14.7%, and the tongue 13.6%. In our material, tumours of the oral cavity occupied the leading position, accounting for up to 59.7% of tumours in the study area. Cancers of the red border of the lips (8.9%), upper jaw (8.3%), and mucosa of the floor of the oral cavity (6.5%) were intermediate in frequency. Rare localisations were mucosal cancer of the alveolar process of the maxilla (3.5%), laryngeal cancer (1.1%), and thyroid cancer (0.5%).

The following regularity was observed in the main and control groups in terms of primary tumour spread: T2 - 12.9% vs. 13.1%, T3 - 28.7% vs. 26.2%, T4 - 58.3% vs. 60.7%, respectively. In the main and control groups in the absolute majority of cases - 87% and 86.9%, respectively, there was a locally spread tumour process.

Regional metastases at the time of treatment were verified in 69 patients (78.8%), of whom 48 (44.4%) in the main group and 21 (34.4%) in the control group. In 98.2% of cases morphologically the tumour was represented by squamous cell cancer, of which orogenic cancer was detected in 59.7% and non-orogenic in 38.4% of cases.

Quality of life parameters before and after were assessed using the Karnofsky scale, 5-point ECOG scale, and EORTC QLQ-H&N-35 questionnaires.

We have developed indications and contraindications to the use of complex vascularised dermofascial and musculoskeletal flaps with axial type of blood circulation depending on the localisation, spread of the tumour process and the category of defect complexity.

Defects formed after surgical interventions were expediently divided into 4 groups: Group I - non-cavitary defects of skin, muscle and bone tissues not communicating with cavities - 36 (21.3%) cases; II группа - несквозные дефекты слизистых оболочек, мышц и костей с сохранными кожными покровами у 115 (68,0%), III категория - сквозные дефекты слизистых оболочек, дефекты мышц и костей, сообщающиеся с поверхностью кожи на большом протяжении - у 13 (7,7%); IV категория дефектов - сквозные дефекты гортани и глотки, т.laryngostomies, pharyngostomies - in 3 (1.7%) patients.

By localisation all defects were divided into 3 groups: Group 1 - defects of the oral cavity and nasal cavities - 111 (65.6%), Group 2 - defects of the skin and soft tissues of the face in 43 (38.5%) patients, Group 3 - defects of the skin of the cranial vault and neck - in 15 (8.9%) patients.

In the main group of patients one-stage reconstruction of defects was performed in 103 (95.3%) cases, delayed plasty - in 5 (4.6%). In the control group of patients in 53 (86,9%) cases after tumour excision the edges of the defect were sutured, and in 8 (13,1%) cases the patients underwent a minimum amount of defect plasty with local tissues and a free split skin flap.

A total of 132 flaps were used to replace postoperative defects, of which 65 (49.2%) were musculoskeletal flaps, of which 37 (56.9%) were represented by a flap of the pectoralis major muscle. Skin-fascial, skin-fat flaps were used in 56 (42.4%) cases, of which 32 (57.1%) were represented by the nasolabial flap and 11 (8.2%) by other types of flaps. In more than 20 (18.5%) cases, combined plasty using more than one flap was performed.

Referring to the results obtained by us, we consider that the most optimal for plasty of non-circumferential defects of the head and neck are skin-fat and skin-fascial flaps, which in our work were used in 56 (42.4%) cases, of which in 32 (57.1%) - was represented by the nasolabial flap. In this regard, we can conclude that the nasolabial skin-fat and skin-fascial flaps have a preferential practical application in reconstructive and restorative head and neck surgery.

A total of 65   (49.2%) were used to replace combined defects in the study area

musculocutaneous flaps, of which the absolute majority of cases n=37 (56.9%) was a flap of the pectoralis major muscle (PMM). This figure is not accidental and once again confirms the data of a number of researchers that despite the improvement of methods of head and neck defect reconstruction and the appearance of new free revascularised flaps, the LGM flap still remains a "workhorse" in head and neck oncosurgery.

Our study also focused on the influence of the volume of surgical intervention on the parameters of patients' quality of life. There were no differences in the initial level of the patients' general condition, their performance, and the quality of life parameters according to the results of the study using specialised scales and questionnaire methods. When statistically analysing the results obtained after the operation, in general, there was a decrease in the severity of the disease symptoms in both groups. However, more significant changes in the quality of life parameters were noted in the main group.

We were able to change the patients' performance status (ECOG) from low to ECOG-0 in 69 (63.9%) patients of the main group and 23 (37.7%) of the control group.

In the studied groups before surgery, the severity of symptoms of malignant tumour: pain sensations, use of analgesics, problem of chewing hard food, missing teeth, trismus of masticatory muscles, feeling of dry mouth and viscosity of saliva, weight loss in patients in both groups before surgery were at the same level. And impaired swallowing, sense of smell, speaking, eating problems in society, social contact and general feeling of sickness were predominant in patients of control group.

After surgery, both groups of patients showed positive changes in the intensity of pain, swallowing, smell and taste disorders, free mouth opening, xerostomia, salivary viscosity, speech, eating in public places, social contact and general feeling of illness. Among the symptoms of the disease, pain, chewing associated with missing teeth were the most disturbing in the main group, while in the control group pain, senses of smell and taste, act of swallowing, missing teeth, problems in social contact in the community and general feeling of sickness were the most disturbing.

In terms of the duration of the operation time the groups were not the same: In the main group on average the operations lasted from 190 to 340 minutes, and in the control group from 120230 minutes, which is due to the one-stage performance of reconstructive-restorative operations in the main group of patients.

We evaluated the results of reconstructive surgeries by complications. A comparative analysis of purulent-necrotic complications of plastic surgeries showed that in the main group their proportion was 37.9%, and in the control group in 34.4% of cases. Partial necrosis of the flap was the most frequent in the main group - 22.2%, and in the control group suture divergence - 31.1%.

The main causes of flap necrosis were a combination of such factors as: previous chemoradiotherapy, which contributed to the formation of fibrosis and impaired regenerative and restorative functions of tissues around the tumour, due to obliteration of blood and lymphatic vessels; impaired rheological properties of patients' blood and microcirculation; reduced nutritional status of patients; fundamentally incorrect flap formation and technical deficiencies - damage to the axial vessel during surgery, compression of the stem of the flap; and the use of the flap as a flap for the treatment of tumour necrosis. **Measures aimed at reducing the incidence of postoperative purulent-necrotic complications in** reconstructive-reconstructive surgeries were provided from the moment of hospitalisation of patients. We have developed criteria for identification and correction of patients at risk of complications. With this in mind, appropriate measures were taken to reduce the risk of complications, affecting different pathogenetic links (stages) of homeostasis.

Thus, at the preoperative stage we evaluated the blood coagulation and anti-coagulation system, 223 cardiovascular system, haemopoiesis and nutritional status of the patients.

As a result, anaemia of moderate and severe degree was diagnosed in 35% of patients, and in 10% of them at moderate severity it was corrected by conservative method with iron-containing preparations, and at severe forms - 25% by haemo- and plasma transfusion on indications.

The nutritional status of the patients was assessed by body mass index (Ketle index) and blood protein composition measured by blood biochemical analysis. In this case, the index of total protein with measurement of serum albumin fraction of blood was assessed.

Before surgery, a body mass index below 19 was diagnosed in 25% of patients in the main group and 20% in the control group.

Hypoproteinaemia, with a decrease in blood albumin fraction was diagnosed in 13% of patients who underwent infusion of 20% solution of human albumin 50.0 ml intravenous drip immediately 2-3 days before surgery.

To improve the rheological properties of blood, we applied solutions of rheopolyglucin, rheosorbilact, Latren 200.0 ml and trental 5.0 ml with dilution on 200.0 ml isotonic solution of 0.9% sodium chloride.

In order to prevent haemorrhage 2-3 hours before the operation, the patients were treated with haemostatic drugs: dicinone - 2.0 ml, epsilon aminocaproic acid - 100.0 ml, ethamsylate sodium - 3.0 ml, tranescamic acid 500 mg - 5.0 ml.

In the postoperative period, standard treatment including infusion, nutritional, antimicrobial, anti-edema and antithrombotic therapy, as well as early activation was performed

patients. To increase blood parameters, 20% of patients also underwent haemo- and plasma transfusion in the postoperative period.

Infusion therapy included normalisation of water-electrolyte and acid-base balance of the patients' organism. For this purpose colloid-crystalloid solutions (Ringer's lactate, haemosol, acesol, trisol) were used as indicated. In order to reduce hypercoagulability and prevent thromboembolic complications, we used direct-acting anticoagulants to maintain blood rheological properties under control of blood clotting time according to Lee-Uwait and Sukharev - heparin (up to 25000-30000 units per day subcutaneously) and its low-molecular fractions - anti-Ha: clexane, fraxiparin, enoxaparin (2000-4000 IU subcutaneously 2-3 times/day), warfarin, as well as solutions that improve blood circulation of the body - reosorbylact, reopolyglucin, trental.

To prevent infectious complications taking into account the sensitivity of flora, we used broad-spectrum antibiotics - 3-4 generation cephalosporins intravenously by 2 g/day, as well as tinidazole derivatives (metronidazole) intravenously by 100 ml x 2 times a day.

It was found that in patients who used haemo-plasmatotransfusion in the perioperative period the incidence of necrosis was 12% higher, which is a motivation to replace blood products with blood substitute solutions.

Postoperative lethality was observed in 2 (1.1%) cases, one case in both groups. The cause of death in one patient was arterial bleeding from the main vessels of the neck and haematoma formation on the 13th day after surgery. The second patient died from bleeding in the early postoperative period on the 1st day.

The immediate functional and cosmetic results of the defects plasty with complex flaps on the pedicle were evaluated and the influence of this type of reconstruction on the quality of life and survival rate of patients with malignant tumours of the head and neck was determined.

During the follow-up period, one-year observed survival in the main and control groups was (96.1% vs. 79.9%), three-year survival was 62.2% vs. 33.7%, and 5-year survival was 33.5% vs. 13.3%.

When comparing the results obtained with the control group, it was noted that the use of one-stage reconstructive-reconstructive surgeries contributes to a decrease in the incidence of recurrences and metastases of the tumour process. This proves the obtained relatively high percentage of overall survival of patients, which, apparently, is achieved by the possibility of wider excision of tumour tissues, thus influencing the radicality of operations.

Our clinical observations and literature data have established that mainly recurrences and metastases of head and neck cancer in most cases occur in the first year after surgery, which is a poor prognostic factor and affects survival. This is confirmed by our data. Thus, the survival rate of patients in the main group after the 1st year to 3 years decreased from 96,1% to 62,2% (difference by 33,9%) and in the control group, this index changed from 79,9% to 33,7% (difference by 46,2%.). Five-year survival rate in the main group was 35.5%, and in the control group - 13.3%, which is 2.7 times less than the main group. The above data allow us to judge about the low survival rate of patients in the control group, which is apparently caused by refusal (abstinence)   from reconstructive surgery.

of the reconstructive stage of surgical treatment, by economical non-radical or conditionally-radical treatment.

(R1 and R2) resections, resulting in a high rate of tumour recurrence and metastasis.

Of the total cohort (169) patients, a total of 209 surgical interventions were performed, of which 1 surgery was performed in 90 and 50 patients in the main and control groups, respectively, 2 surgeries in 11 and 8 patients, 3 surgeries in 6 and 3 patients, and 4 surgeries in 1 patient in the main group (Table 59).

Table 59. - Total number of operations in the main and the control group

Number of operations	Main group	Total number of	Control group	Total number of
1 operation	90 (83,3%)	90	50 (82,0%)	**50**
2 operations	11 (10,2%)	22	8 (13,1%)	**16**
3 operations	6 (5,5%)	18	3 (4,1%)	**9**
4 operations	1 (0,9%)	4	-	-
Total	**108**	**134**	**61**	**75**

The question of the sequence of radiotherapy and surgery remains relevant and debatable both in the literature and in our practice. In our study in both groups of patients who received neoadjuvant radiotherapy and chemoradiotherapy complications were noted twice as often (26.6% vs. 13.5%), which dictates the need to perform at the first stage surgical intervention before chemoradiotherapy.

The analysis of the available literature and our own clinical material on the problem of the possibility of performing one-stage reconstructive-restorative surgeries as the first stage of combined and complex treatment of locally advanced squamous cell carcinoma of the head and neck organs allow us to draw the following **conclusions:**

- It was found that the most frequent defects were localised in the oral and nasal cavities - 61.1%, face - 29.6%, skull vault and neck - 9.3% *(p = 0.096)*. Predominantly the defects were represented by category II and I of complexity (68.6% and 21.3%, respectively).

- The analysis of head and neck defects reconstruction methods revealed that in the main group one-stage flap plasty was performed in 95.4%, delayed - in 4.6% of cases, the most frequently used flaps were musculoskeletal - 65 (49.2%), skin-fat and skin-fascial - 56 (42.4%). In 18.5% of cases, defect plasty was combined.

- In oral cavity defects (II-III category) n = 66 (61,1%) the optimal method of plasty is skin-muscular (BGM - 43,0%, PPL - 15,2%) and skin-fascial (DFL - 11,4%) grafts and a combination of two or more flaps. In facial defects (I-II categories) n=32 (29.6%) - skin-fat and skin-fascial flaps (NGL - 34.1%), and in skin defects of the cranial vault and neck (I, II, IV categories) n=10 (9.3%) - skin-fat, skin-fascial and flaps and free skin grafts.

- An algorithm for monitoring the immediate postoperative period and prevention of postoperative complications was developed and applied, which contributed to a 16.5% reduction in complications in the prospective group (p=0.083).

- Good perception of the results of reconstructive-restorative surgeries in functional and aesthetic terms was greater in the main group than in the control group (32.4% and 18.5% vs. 3.3% and 3.3%; p < 0.05). Unsatisfactory perception of results was less in the main group than in the control group (3.7% 6.5% vs. 13.1% and 18.0%; p < 0.05).

- Reconstructive-restorative surgeries improved the quality of life in the main group in 63.9% of patients according to ECOG status and Karnofsky index (p < 0.01). In the same group, 1-, 3- and 5-year observed survival rates improved - 96.1%, 62.2% and 33.5%, respectively (p <0.001).

The obtained results of our own clinical studies can be accepted for implementation in practical healthcare (oncology, plastic surgery) in the form of the **following recommendations:**

- One-stage reconstructive-reconstructive surgery of defects after removal of the defect locally

The use of arterialised flaps for advanced head and neck cancer should become an obligatory stage that improves the quality of life of patients, speeds up their rehabilitation and hospital stay.

- In the presence of resectable head and neck cancer, adequate surgical intervention with defect reconstruction at the first stage is recommended, which contributes not only to reducing the incidence of postoperative complications, but also improves the quality of life and accelerates postoperative rehabilitation of patients.

- Musculoskeletal and dermofascial flaps with axial circulation alone and in combination have proven to be the best plastic material and can be an alternative to microsurgical flaps, especially in resource-limited settings.

- At the stage of preoperative preparation it is necessary to divide patients into subgroups, taking into account the localisation and characteristics of the defect formed, which allows choosing the most optimal flap for their replacement without additional loss of time in the operating theatre.

- It is advisable to start measures for the prevention of postoperative complications from the moment of patients' admission to the hospital and to accompany them in all stages of surgical treatment.

- Functional and aesthetic results should be assessed in conjunction with the patients, taking into account their subjective perceptions of the results obtained.

REFERENCE LIST

1. Analysis of 10-year experience of treatment and rehabilitation of patients with malignant skin tumours of the head and neck in Moscow / A. M. Sdvizhkov [et al.] // Siberian Oncological Journal. - 2012. - №4,- C. 84-85.

2. Badalyan A. G. Surgical treatment of locally advanced recurrent skin cancer of the external ear. Case from practice / A. G. Badalyan, A. M. Mudunov // Head and Neck Tumours. - 2013. - №3. - C. 43-46.

3. Possibilities of nasolabial flap in facial reconstructive surgery / U. A. Kurbanov [et al. A. Kurbanov [et al] // Vestnik Avicenna. - 2008. № 3.- C.9 19.

4. Possibilities of reconstruction of oral cavity defects with the nasolabial flap / Sh.I. Musin [et al] // Eurasian Journal of Oncology. - 2016. - T. 4, № 2. - C. 150-151.

5. Restoration of sound formation and speech in cancer patients with defects of the upper jaw / Kulakov A.A.. [et al.] // Tumours of the head and neck. - 2012. - №1. - C. 55-59.

6. Choice of surgical treatment option for recurrent cancer of oropharyngeal organs / Zaderenko I.A. [et al. [et al.] // Head and Neck Tumours. -2017.-T. 7, № 2. - C. 25-29.

7. Vyrupaev S.V. Improvement of the results of surgical rehabilitation of patients with neoplasms and defects of the head and neck: Cand. Dr. of medical sciences. / S.V. Vyrupaev. - Ufa, 2005. - 346 c.

8. Davydov M.I. Statistics of malignant neoplasms in Russia and CIS countries in 2012 / M.I. Davydov, E.M. Axel. - Moscow: Izd. group RONC, 2014. - 226 c.

9. Dashkova, I. R. Reconstructive and plastic surgeries in the complex treatment of patients with locally advanced superficial tumours / Dashkova I. R., Irkhina A. N. // VII Congress of Oncologists of Russia. N. // VII Congress of Oncologists of Russia. Scientific and practical conference with international participation. Collection of materials. Volume H.-M.-2009, -C.185.

10. Organ-preserving treatment of squamous cell carcinoma of oropharyngeal area with determination of individual prognosis of radiotherapy efficacy / A.R. Gevorkov // Eurasian Journal of Oncology. - 2016. - T. 4, № 2.- C. 111.

11. Zeynalova S.M. Treatment of locally advanced primary and recurrent squamous cell carcinoma of the head and neck skin / S.M. Zeynalova, N.M. Amiraliev // Medical News. - 2016. - №5. - C. 62-64.

12. Malignant tumours of the tongue - surgical treatment. The golden rule in the choice of reconstructive material. Creating optimal rehabilitation conditions / Pismenny [et al.] // Eurasian Journal of Oncology. - 2016. - №2. - C. 52-52.

13. Ivanova O.V. Justification of complex therapy of stomatological diseases in patients with locally spread cancer of the oral cavity mucosa: Cand. Doctor of medical sciences / O.V. Ivanova. - Saratov, 2016. - 218 c.

14. Ignatova A.V. Prognostic value of biomarkers in oral squamous cell cancer. Literature review / A. V. Ignatova, A. M. Mudunov, M. N. Narimanov // Tumours of the head and neck.-2014.- №4.-P.28-33.

15. The use of free radial flap for the replacement of complex postoperative defects in combined and complex treatment of patients with locally advanced squamous cell cancer of the oral cavity / Chen X. [et al.] // Head and Neck Tumours. - 2020. - T. 10, №1. - C. 55-64.

16. Caprin, A.D. Malignant neoplasms in Russia in 2018 (morbidity and mortality) / A.D. Caprin, V.V. Starinsky, G.V. Petrova. Starinsky, G.V. Petrova. - Moscow: P.A. Herzen MNIOI, 2019. - 250 c.

17. Kaprin A.D., Malignant neoplasms in Russia in 2019 (morbidity and mortality). AD. Kaprin, V.V. Starinsky, A.O. Shakhzadova. - Moscow: P.A. Herzen MNIOI - a branch of FGBU "NMRC Radiology" of the Ministry of Health of Russia, 2020. - ill. - 252 c.

18. Clinical case of successful application of pembrolizumab in the treatment of recurrent inoperable squamous cell carcinoma of the head and neck / Mudunov A.M. [et al.] // 232
Tumours of the head and neck. - 2019. - T. 9, № 1. - C. 93-98.

19. Klipka, A.I. Oral mucosal cancer, the possibilities of primary surgical rehabilitation of patients in complex treatment / A.I. Klipka // Eurasian Journal of Oncology. - 2016. - T. 4, № 2. - C. 118.

20. Klipka A.I. Choice of mandibular resection volume in surgical treatment of oral mucosa cancer / A.I. Klipka [et al.] // Eurasian Journal of Oncology. - 2016. - T. 4, № 2. - C. 129.

21. Combined immunotargeted therapy with nivolumab and cetuximab:

new opportunities in the treatment of head and neck squamous cell cancer / A. M. Mudunov [et al.] // Head and Neck Tumours. - 2020. - T. 10, № 3. - C. 111-17.

22. Kutukova S.I. Modern approaches to the choice of therapy for locally advanced and recurrent/metastatic squamous cell carcinoma of the head and neck: what is the rationale for the choice of therapy in clinical practice? / S.I.Kutukova // Pharmateka. - 2018. - №7. - C. 50-56.

23. Makarevich M.N. Application of free radial flap in surgical rehabilitation of patients with tongue cancer / M.N. Makarevich, I.V. Belotserkovsky // Eurasian Journal of Oncology. - 2016. - T. 4, № 2. - C.141-42.

24. Matyakin E. G. G. Reconstructive surgeries for head and neck tumours / E. G. Matyakin. - Moscow: Berdana, 2009. - 224 c.

25. Microsurgical reconstruction of the hard palate after resections for malignant tumours / M. V. Bolotin [et al.] // Head and Neck Tumours. - 2020. - VOL. 10, № 4.-P.25 -31.

26. Minaylo I.I. Long-term results of treatment of patients suffering from locally advanced cancer
oropharyngeal zone / I.I. Minaylo, A.R. Ekshembeeva, N.A. Artemova // Eurasian Journal of Oncology. - 2016. - T. 4, № 2.-C.136-37.

27. Mudunov AM. Human papillomavirus - a new etiological factor in the development of head and neck cancer. Problems and prospects for their solution / AM. Mudunov // Epidemiology and vaccine prophylaxis. - 2018. - T. 17, №5. - C. 100-6.

28. Mudunov A. M. Correction of nutritional deficiency in patients with squamous cell carcinoma of the oropharyngeal zone / A. M. Mudunov, D. B. Udintsov // Head and Neck Tumours. - 2015. - T. 5, № 3.-C.13-15.

29. Mudunov A. M. Nutritional support of patients during surgical treatment of squamous cell carcinoma of the oral cavity mucosa / A. M. Mudunov, D. B. Udintsov // Head and Neck Tumours. - 2017. - T. 7, № 3. - C. 47-52.

30. Mudunov AM. Nivolumab in the treatment of refractory recurrent and metastatic squamous cell carcinoma of head and neck organs. Results of the clinical trial of phase III CHECKMATE 141 / A.M.

Mudunov // Head and Neck Tumours. - 2017. - T. 7, № 3. - C. 74-86.

31. Mudunov A. M. New possibilities of immunotherapy in the treatment of advanced recurrent squamous cell carcinoma of head and neck organs / A. M. Mudunov, M. N. Narimanov, D. A. Safarov // Head and Neck Tumours. - 2017. - T. 7, № 2. - C. 99 - 105.

32. Mudunov, A. M. / Long-term results of treatment of patients with locally advanced skin cancer of the external ear / A. M. Mudunov, E. G. Khazarova, M. V. Bolotin // Tumours of the head and neck. - 2021.-T.il, №1.-C.12-23.

33. Mudunov AM. Endolaryngeal laser resections of the larynx / A.M. Mudunov, M.V. Bolotin // Tumours of the head and neck. -2016.-T. 6, NO. H.-P. 34-37.

34. Mudunov A. M. Effectiveness of modern methods of treatment of locally advanced skin cancer of the external ear: a review of the literature / A. M. Mudunov, E. G. Khazarova, Y. V. Alymov // Head and Neck Tumours. - 2020. - T. 10, № 4. - C. 86-90.

35. Review of the possibilities of regional intraarterial chemotherapy in the treatment of squamous cell carcinoma of the nasal cavity and sinuses / A.M. Mudunov [et al]. // Head and Neck Tumours. - 2018. - T. 8, №1. - C. 56-61.

36. Oncology. Clinical Recommendations. / Edited by Acad. of RAS M.I. Davydov. - Moscow: RONC Publishing Group, 2015. - 680 c.

37. Oncology: A guide to clinical oncology.

Part-3. Reconstructive surgeries and modern methods of treatment of solitary and primary-multiple tumours of maxillofacial region and neck / edited by N.I. Bazarov. - Dushanbe, "Sharqi ozod", 2018. - 560 c.

38. Osipyan E. O. Computed and magnetic resonance imaging in the assessment of local prevalence of oral cavity and oropharynx tumours as a major factor in the choice of treatment tactics (literature review) / E. O. Osipyan, A. M. Mudunov // Head and Neck Tumours. - 2017. T. 7, №4. C. 53-62.

39. Assessment of quality of life in palliative care / G.A. Novikov [et al]. - Ulyanovsk: Ul'yanovsk State University, 2013. -114 c.

40. Assessment of the quality of life of patients with advanced oral mucosa cancer after surgery using microsurgical plasty / AV. Karpenko [et al.] // Eurasian Journal of Oncology. - 2016. - T. 4, № 2. - C. 106-7.

41. Assessment of psychosomatic status in providing palliative care to cancer patients / D.F.Ganiev [et al.] // Bulletin of the Academy of Medical Sciences of Tajikistan. - 2O17.- № 2.- PP.10-15.

42. Paches A.I. Tumours of the head and neck: Clinical Manual / A.I. Paches. - 5th ed., revised and supplemented. - M.: Practical Medicine, 2013. - 478 c.

43. Pismenny V.I. Speech therapy after surgical treatment of malignant tumours of the oropharyngeal zone / V.I. Pismenny, N.M. Kulakova, I.V. Pismenny // Proceedings of the Samara Scientific Centre of the Russian Academy of Sciences. - 2015. - T. 17, № 2. - C. 622 - 27.

44. Pismenny V.I. Topographo-anatomical justification of the use of skin-muscular flap with thyroid artery for reconstructive surgeries in the oropharyngeal region / V.I. Pismenny, S.N. Chemidronov, I.V. Pismenny // Eurasian Journal of Oncology. - 2016. - №2. - C. 52-53.

45. Pismenny V.I. Extirpation of the tongue. Issues of rehabilitation / V.I. Pismenny, N.M. Kulakova, I.V. Pismenny // Eurasian Journal of Oncology. - 2016. - T. 4,-№2.C.55-56.

46. Practical recommendations for the treatment of malignant tumours of the head and neck / L.V.Bolotina [et al] // Malignant tumours: Practical recommendations RUSSCO, - 2017. -T.7.- P. 66-76.

47. Principles of radiotherapy of laryngeal cancer / Alieva S. B.. [et al.] // Head and neck tumours. - 2021. - T. 11, №1. - C. 24-33.

48. Positron emission tomography with 18F-fluorodeoxyglucose combined with computed tomography in head and neck squamous cell cancer (literature review) / Ryzhova O. D. Д. [et al.] // Tumours of the head and neck. - 2019.- VOL. 9, NO. 3, PP. 49-60.

49. Postoperative complications in combined treatment of locally advanced and recurrent oropharyngeal cancer / Sikorsky D.V.. [et al.] Tumours of the head and neck. - 2014. - № 3,- C. 40-46.

50. Psychological distress in cancer patients after laryngectomy / Tkachenko G. A.. [et al.] // Tumours of the head and neck. - 2019. - T.9. №1. - C. 104-110.

51. Psychological assistance to patients after laryngectomy / Tkachenko G. A.. [et al.] // Tumours of the head and neck. - 2020. - T.10. №1. - C. 101-106.

52. Psychosomatic state of patients before and after correction of

maxillofacial defects by orthopaedic method / A. A. Akhundov. [et al.] // Head and Neck Tumours. - 2012. - №4. - C. 40-45.

53. Reconstruction of full-thickness defects of the cheek region after tumour removal using a modified technique of submental flap taking / Ch.R. Rahimov [et al.] // Head and Neck Tumours. - 2018. - T. 8, № 2. - C.27-33.

54. Reconstructive-plastic operations in patients with malignant neoplasms of the tongue, mucosa of the floor of the oral cavity, types of plastic surgery / Z.A. Rajabova [et al.] // Head and Neck Tumours. - 2015. - №1. - C.15 -18.

55. Oral mucosa cancer - two sides of the same problem / G.A. Ginzburg [et al.] // Siberian Oncological Journal. - 2010. - T. 39, № 3. - C. 61-62.

56. Rehabilitation of oncological patients with defect and complete secondary adentia after removal of both upper jaws / Kulakov A.A. // Head and Neck Tumours. - 2012. - №4. - C. 34-39.

57. Regional intra-arterial polychemotherapy as a method of increasing the effectiveness of conservative treatment of locally advanced squamous cell carcinoma of the oral cavity mucosa / AM.Mudunov [et al]. // Tumours of the head and neck. - 2019. - T.9, №3. C. 24-28. '

58. Results of using free osteomyofascial grafts for one-stage reconstruction of combined postresection facial defects with intraoral component / Sharapo A. S. [et al.] // Head and Neck Tumours. - 2020. - T. 10, № 2. - C. 22-29.

59. Results of conservative treatment of locally disseminated local squamous cell laryngeal cancer by intra-arterial regional application of polychemotherapy / Safarov D. A.. [et al.] // Head and Neck Tumours. - 2021. - T.H. №1. C. 41-50.

60. Reconstructive and reconstructive operations in surgery of locally advanced malignant tumours of the head and neck / V.S. Protsyk [et al.] // Clinical Oncology. - 2O11.-№ 1. C.1-5.

61. Rhinoplasty for posttraumatic nasal deformities / U. A. Kurbanov [et al. A. Kurbanov [et al] // Avicenna Bulletin. - 2008. № 2. - C. 1322.

62. The role and significance of randomisation in scientific medical research / Sh.Z. Habibulaev [et al.] // Eurasian Journal of Oncology. - 2017. - T. 5, № 1, - C. 81-86.

63. The role of periodontopathogens in carcinogenesis of squamous cell carcinoma of the oral cavity mucosa / A. E. Kazimov [et al.] Tumours of the head and neck. - 2020. - T. 10, № 4. - C. 74 - 85.

64. Romanov, I.S. Early stages of oral cancer. The problem of treatment volume selection / I.S. Romanov, I.M. Gelfand, D.B. Udintsov // Eurasian Journal of Oncology. - 2016. - T. 4, № 2.-C.125.

65. Saprina O.A. Supraclavicular flap in the reconstruction of head and neck defects (literature review) / O.A. Saprina, R.I. Azizyan, Lomaya M.V. // Head and Neck Tumours. - 2017. - T. 7, №1. - C. 46-49.

66. Method of treatment of locally advanced tongue root cancer / Zaderenko I. A.. [et al.] // Head and Neck Tumours. - 2018. -T. 8, № 1. - C.12-16.

67. Tkachenko, G.A. Clinical and psychological study of the quality of life of patients suffering from malignant neoplasms of the maxillofacial region / G.A. Tkachenko // Bulletin of Psychotherapy. - 2012. - T. 44. - C. 57-63.

68. Transoral laser resections of tumours of the oral cavity and oropharynx / M. V. Bolotin [et al.] // Head and Neck Tumours. - 2016.-№1.-C.28-32.

69. Uklonskaya, D.V. Speech restoration in acquired anatomical defects and deformations of the maxillofacial region / D.V. Uklonskaya. Moscow: Logomag, 2017. -104 c.

70.   Functional results of application Subclavian skin-muscular flap for plasty of oncological defects of the oral cavity / A. V. Karpenko [et al.] // Malignant tumours. - 2016. - T. 17, №1. - C. 36-43.

71. Khabibulaev Sh.Z. Long-term results of surgical treatment of locally advanced head and neck cancer / Sh.Z. Khabibulaev / Vestnik Avicenna. - 2010. -№1.- C. 44-49.

72. Khabibulaev Sh.Z. Reconstructive and reconstructive operations at locally spread cancer of the head and neck organs: Cand. Dr. of medical sciences / Sh.Z. Habibulaev. - Rostov-on-Don, 2011.-229 p.

73. Khodjamuradov G.M. Choice of reconstruction method in posttraumatic defects of nerve trunks / G.M. Khodjamuradov, K.P. Artykov // Bulletin of Ivanovo Medical Academy. - 2012. - T. 17, № 4. - C. 63-68.

74. Chissov V.I. Oncology. National Manual / ed. by V.I. Chisov, M.I. Davydov. - Moscow: GEOTAR-Media, 2017. - 624 c.

75. A comparison between the pectoralis major myocutaneous flap and thefreeanterolateralalthigh perforator flap for reconstruction in head and neck cancer patients: assessment of the quality of life *I* X. Zhang [et al.] // J Craniofac Surg. - 2014. - V. 25. - N.3.- P. 868-71.

76. Aesthetic Outcome After Reconstruction of Complex Soft Tissue Defects with Free Antero-Lateral Thigh Flap Using Simple Equipment *I* A. H. Abbas [et al.] // Journal of Surgery. - 2015. - V.3. - N. 2. - P. 3641.

77. AJCC Cancer Staging Manual, ed 8. *I* M.B. Amin [et al]. - New York.: Springer International Publishing, - 2017. - 1032 p.

78. An international phase 3 trial in head and neck cancer: quality of life and symptom results: EORTC Head and Neck and the EORTC Radiation Oncology Group *I* A. Bottomley [et al.] // Cancer. - 2014. - V. 120.-N. 3.-P.390-98.

79. Anicin, A. Pectoralis Major Myocutaneous Flap in Primary and Salvage Head and Neck Cancer Surgery *I* A. Anicin, R. Sifrer, P. Strojan // Journal of Oral and Maxillofacial Surgery. - 2015. - V. 73. - № 10. - P. 2057-64.

80. An update on head and neck squamous cell carcinoma in respect to classification and systemic therapy *I* A.M. Mudunov [et al.] // Head and Neck Tumors. - 2018. -V. 8. -N.I.- P. 48-55.

81. Ariyan S. The pectoralis major myocutaneous flap: A versatile flap for reconstruction in the head and neck *I* S. Ariyan *II* Plastic and Reconstructive Surgery. -1979. - V. 63, № 1. - P. 73-81.

82. Assessment of the quality of life of patients with oral cancer after pectoralis major myocutaneous flap reconstruction with a focus on speech *I* Q. G. Fang [et al.] // Journal of Oral and Maxillofacial Surgery. - 2013. - V. 71. - N. 11. - P. 2004.el-e5.

83. Atlas of regional and free flaps for head and neck reconstruction: flap harvest and insetting *I* Mark L Urken .... [et al.]; illustrator, Sharon Ellis. - 2nd ed. - 2012, 549 pg.

84. Bakamjian, V.Y. A two-stage method for pharyngoesophageal reconstruction with a primary pectoral skin flap *I NX.* Bakamjian // Plast Reconstr Surg. - 1965. - V. 36. - P. 173-84.

85. Bannister, M., Ah-See, K. W. Enhanced recovery programmes in head and neck surgery: systematic review / M. Bannister [et al.] // The Journal of Laryngology & Otology. - 2015. - V. 129. - N. 5. - P. 416-20.

86. Best practices in the management of the psycho-oncologic aspects of head and neck cancer patients: recommendations from the European Head and Neck Cancer Society Make Sense Campaign / M. Reich [et al.] // Ann Oncol. - 2014. - V. 25. - N.ll. - P. 2115-24.

87. Burden of HPV-positive oropharynx cancers among ever and never smokers in the U.S. population / Chaturvedi P. [et al.] // Oral Oncol. - 2016. - V. 60. - P. 61-67.

88. Comparison of Oral Function: Free Anterolateral Thigh Perforator Flaps Versus Vascularised Free Forearm Flap for Reconstruction in Patients Undergoing Glossectomy / Y. Yuan [et al.] // J Oral Maxillofac Surg. - 2016. - V. 74. -N.7.- P. 1500el-e6.

89. Daniel R.K.. Distant transfer of an island flap by microvascular anastomoses. A clinical technique / R.K. Daniel, G.I. Taylor //Plast Reconstr Surg. - 1973. - V. 52. -N.2.- P. 111-17.

90. Development of the Pectoral Perforator Flap and the Deltopectoral Perforator Flap Pedicled with the Pectoralis Major Muscle Flap /Y. Nishi [et al.] // Annals of Plastic Surgery. - 2013. - V. 71.-N. 4.-P. 365-71.

91. Djan R. A systematic review of questionnaires to measure the impact of appearance on quality of life for head and neck cancer patients / R. Djan, A. Penington //J. Plastic, Reconstructive & Aesthetic Surgery. - 2013. - V. 66. -N.5.- P. 647-59.

92. Economic analyses in squamous cell carcinoma of the head and neck: a review of the literature from a clinical perspective / J.A. De Souza [et al.] // Int J Radiat Oncol Biol Phys. - 2014. - V. 89. - N.5. - P. 989-96.

93. Estimating the global cancer incidence and mortality in 2018: GLOBOCAN sources and methods / J. Ferlay [et al] // Int Journal of Cancer. - 2019. - V. 144. - N.8.- P. 1941-53.

94. Extended vertical lower trapezius island myocutaneous flap versus pectoralis major myocutaneous flap for reconstruction in recurrent oral and oropharyngeal cancer / W.L. Chen [et al.] // Head & Neck. - 2016. - V. 38. - Suppl. 1. - P. E159-64.

95. EUROGIN roadmap: comparative epidemiology of HPV infection and associated cancers of the head and neck and cervix / M.L. Gillison [et al.] //Int J Cancer. - 2014. - V. 134. - N. 3. - P. 497507.

96. Factors affecting wound complications in head and neck surgery: A prospective study / A. Deshmukh [et al.] // Indian Journal of Medical and Paediatric Oncology. - 2013. - V. 34. - N. 4. - P. 24751.

97. Functional lower lip reconstruction with the modified Bernard-Webster flap / R. Denadai [et al.] // J. of Plastic, Reconstructive and Aesthetic Surgery. - 2015. - V. 68. - N. 11. - P. tr2-28.

98. Goldwyn, R.M. An experimental study of large island flaps in dogs / R.M. Goldwyn, D.L. Lamb, W.L. White // Plast Reconstr Surg. - 1963.-V.31.-P.528-36.

99. Harashina, T. Reconstruction of the oral cavity with a free flap / T. Harashina, T. Fujino, F. Aoyagi // Plast Reconstr Surg. - 1976. - V. 58.-N. 4.-P. 412-14.

100. Harii K. Successful clinical transfer of ten flaps by microvascular anastomoses / K. Harii, K. Omori, S. Omori // Plast Reconstr Surg. - 1974. - V. 53. -N.3.- P. 259-70.

101. Head and Neck cancer: improving outcomes with a multidisciplinary approach / C. Lo Nigro [et al.] // Cancer manag Res. - 2017.-V. 9.-P. 363-71

102. Head and Neck Cancer. NCCN Clinical Practice Guidelines in Oncology, ver. 1. 2021. - 219 p.

103. Head and neck cancer patients' quality of life / K.H. Nelke [et al.] // Adv Clin Exp Med. - 2014. -V.23.-N.6.- P. 1019-27.

104. Head and neck cancer prevention: from primary prevention to impact of clinicians on reducing burden / D. Hashim [et al] // Ann Oncol. - 2019. - V. 30. -N. 5.- P. 744-56.

105. Head and neck cancer surgery in an elderly patient population: a retrospective review / R. Yang [et al.] // International Journal of Oral and Maxillofacial Surgery. - 2014. -. V. 43. - N.12. - P. 1413-17.

106. Head and Neck Reconstruction by Using Extended Pectoralis Major Myocutaneous Flap / S. Azumi [et al.] // J. of Reconstructive Microsurgery. - 2015. - V. 31, № 4. - P. 300-304.

107. Head and neck squamous cell carcinoma / D. E. Johnson [et al.] // Nature Reviews Disease Primers. - 2020. -V.6.- N. 1. - P. 1-22.

108. Health-related quality of life before and after head and neck squamous cell carcinoma: Analysis of the Surveillance, Epidemiology, and End Results-Medicare Health Outcomes Survey linkage *I* E.M.. Rettig [et al] *11* Cancer. - 2016. - V. 122. - N. 12. - P. 1861-70.

109. Hemifacial reimplantation in surgical treatment of maxillary sinus cancer: a case report *I* *I*.V. Reshetov [et al.] //Annals of Oral & Maxillofacial Surgery. - 2013. - V. 20. -N.3.- P. 1-7.

110. Induction chemotherapy followed by concurrent radiochemotherapy versus concurrent radio-chemotherapy alone as treatment of locally advanced squamous cell carcinoma of the head and neck: A meta-analysis of randomised trials IW. Budach [et al.] // Radiotherapy and Oncology. - 2016. - V. 118. -N.2.- P. 238-43.

111. *Iqbal* H. Image guided surgery in the management of head and neck cancer *I* H. Iqbal, Q. Pan // Oral Oncology. Pan // Oral Oncology. - 2016. - V. 57. - P. 32-39.

112. Janis J. E. The New Reconstructive Ladder: Modifications to the Traditional Model. Plastic and Reconstructive Surgery *I* J.E. Janis, R.K. Kwon, C.E.Attinger, *11* - 2011. - V. 127. - P. 205-12.

113. Jatin Shah's Head and Neck Surgery and Oncology, 5th Edition, Elsevier publ., 2019, 896 p.

114. Jensen R.E.. Assessing health-related quality of life in cancer trials *I* R.E. Jensen, C.M. Moinpour, D.L. Fairclough // Clin Invest. - 2012. -. V. 2.-N.6.-P.563-77.

115. Khundkar R. The coracoid process is supplied by a direct branch of the 2nd part of the axillary artery permitting the use of the coracoid as a vascularised bone flap, and improving it's viability in Latarjet or Bristow procedures *I* R. Khundkar, H. Giele // Journal of Plastic, Reconstructive and Aesthetic Surgery. - 2019. - V. 72. - № 4. - P. 609-15.

116. Kim E. K. Method to help ensure survival of a very small skin paddle of pectoralis major musculocutaneous flap in head and neck reconstruction *I* E.K. Kim, S.J. Yang, S.H. Choi // Head & Neck. - 2013. -V. 35.-N. 8.-P. 237-39.

117. Klussmann J.P. Head and neck cancer - New insights into a heterogeneous disease *I* J. P. Klussmann // Oncol Res Treat. - 2017. - V.40.-N. 6.-P.3133-96

118. Lam S. M. Fat Grafting for Facial Contouring *I* S.M. Lam // Facial Plastic Surgery. - 2019. - V. 35. -N.3.- P. 278-85.

119. Lessons Learned from Unfavourable Microsurgical Head and Neck Reconstruction *IY*. Kimata [et al.] // Clinics in Plastic Surgery. - 242

2016. - V. 43. - P. 4. - P. 729-737.

120. Licitra L. Individualised quality of life as a measure to guide treatment choices in squamous cell carcinoma of the head and neck *I* L. Licitra, R. Mesia, U. Keilholz // Oral Oncology. - 2016. - V. 52. - P. 18-23.

121. Lundbech M. Prevalence of venous thromboembolism following head and neck cancer surgery: A systematic review and meta-analysis *I* M. Lundbech, A.E. Krag, A.M. Hvas // Thrombosis Research. - 2018. - V. 169. - P. 30-34.

122. Marur Sh. Head and Neck Squamous Cell Carcinoma: Update on Epidemiology, Diagnosis, and Treatment *I* Sh. Marur, A.A. Forastiere // Mayo Clin Proc. - 2016 - V. 91. -N.3.- P. 386-96.

123. Maxillary Sinus Squamous Cell Carcinoma: A Clinical Study *I* N. Hohchi [et al.] // Int J Pract Otolaryngology. - 2018. №1. - P. elO- el5.

124. Mitchell, O. Rehabilitation of patients following major head and neck cancer surgery *I* O. Mitchell, A. Durrani, R. Price // British Journal of Nursing // British Journal of Nursing. Mitchell, A. Durrani, R. Price // British Journal of Nursing. - 2012. - V. 13. - N. 21. - P. S31-S37.

125. Morris M, Unhold G. Use of flaps in reconstructive surgery of the head and neck. LJ P. Principle of Oral and Maxillofacial Surgery. Philadelphia, Pa: Lippincott; 1992. 947 p.

126. Multivariate analysis of risk factors for postoperative wound infection following oral and oropharyngeal cancer surgery *I* M. Belusic-Gobic [et al.] // Journal of Cranio-Maxillofacial Surgery. - 2018. - V. 46. - N.I. - P. 135-41.

127. NCCN Guidelines Insights: Head and Neck Cancers, Version 1.2018. *I* A.D. Colevas [et al.] // Journal of the National Comprehensive Cancer Network. - 2018. - V. 16. -N.5.- P. 479-90.

128. NCCN Clinical Practice Guidelines: Head and Neck Cancers. Version 1.2018 *I* Pfister D. G. [et al.] // Journal of the National Comprehensive Cancer Network. - 2018. - 218 p.

129. O'Brien BM. Replantation and reconstructive microvascular surgery. Part *11* B. O'Brien // Ann R Coll Surg Engl. - 1976. - V. 58. - N. 2.-P. 87-103.

130. Panje, W.R.. Reconstruction of the oral cavity with a free flap.Plast Reconstr Surg *1* W.R. Panje, J. Bardach, C.J. Krause // - 1976. Krause // - 1976. - V. 58. -N.4.- P. 415-18.

131. Pectoralis major myocutaneous flap in head and neck reconstruction: An experience in 100 consecutive cases *1* M. Tripathi [et al.] // Natl J Maxillofac Surg. -2015.-V. 6. -N. 1. - P. 37-41.

132. Palliative surgery for head and neck cancer with extensive skin involvement *1* D. W. Jang [et al.] // The Laryngoscope. - 2013. - V. 123.-N.5.-P.1173-77.

133. Patel K. Pectoralis major myocutaneous flap *1* K. Patel, D. J.-H Lyu, D. Kademani // Oral and Maxillofacial Surgery Clinics of North America. - 2014. - V. 26. -N.3.- P. 421-26.

134. Patient perception of speech outcomes: the relationship between clinical measures and self-perception of speech function following surgical treatment for oral cancer *1* G. Constantinescu [et al] American J Speech-Lang Pathology. - 2017. - V. 26. - N. 2. - P. 241-47.

135. Pectoralis Major Myocutaneous Flap - Still a Workhorse for Maxillofacial Reconstruction in Developing Countries *1* K. S. Gadre [et al.] // Journal of Oral and Maxillofacial Surgery. - 2013. - V. 11. - N. 71.-P.2005.el-el0.

136. Pectoralis major myofascial only and myocutaneous flaps and pharyngocutaneous fistula in salvage laryngectomy *1* M. R. Gilbert [et al.] // The Laryngoscope. - 2014. - V. 124. - N. 12. - P. 2680-86.

137. Pei S. Application of pectoralis major myocutaneous flap to reconstruction of defects in head and neck cancer *1* S. Pei, L. Xue, X. Wang // Lin Chung Er Bi Yan Hou Tou Jing Wai Ke Za Zhi. - 2013. - V. 27. - N. 12. - P. 667-8. Chinese.

138. Petti S. Alcohol is not a risk factor for oral cancer in nonsmoking, betel quid non-chewing individuals. A metaanalysis update *1* S. Petti, M. Masood, G.A. Messano // Annali di Igiene. - 2013. -V. 25.-N. l.-P. 3-14.

139. Prevalence of human papillomavirus in oropharyngeal and nonoropharyngeal head and neck cancer-systematic review and meta-analysis of trends by time and region *1* Mehanna H [et al.] *11* Head

Neck. - 2013. - V. 35. - P. 747-55.

140. Prevention and management of bacterial infections of the donor site of flaps raised for reconstruction in head and neck surgery / M. Zirk [et al.] // Journal of Cranio-Maxillofacial Surgery. - 2018. - V. 46. - N. 9. - P. 1669-73.

141. Quality of life, cognitive, physical and emotional function at diagnosis predicts head and neck cancer survival: analysis of cases from the Head and Neck 5000 study / S.N. Roger [et al.] // Eur Arch Otorhinolaryngol. - 2020. - V. 277. - P. 1515-23.

142. Radial forearm free flap for reconstruction of the oral cavity: clinical experience in 55 cases / R. Gonzalez-Garcia [et al.] // Oral Surgery, Oral Medicine, Oral Pathology, Oral Radiology, and Endodontology. - 2007. - V. 104. -N.I.- P. 29-37.

143. Reconstruction of advance head and neck cancer patients after tumour ablation with simultaneous multiple free flaps: Indications and prognosis / S. H. Chien [etal.] // Annals of Plastic Surgery. - 2012. - V. 69.-N. 6.-P. 611-15.

144. Reconstruction of Complex Facial Defects Using Cervical Expanded Flap Prefabricated by Temporoparietal Fascia Flap / L. Zhang [et al.] // Journal of Craniofacial Surgery. - 2015. - V. 26. -. N. 6. - P.e472-75.

145. Regional Flaps in Head and Neck Reconstruction: A Reappraisal / G. Colletti [et al.] // Journal of Oral and Maxillofacial Surgery. - 2015. - V. 73. -N.3.- P. 571.el-10.

146. Resection and reconstruction of giant cervical metastatic cancer using a pectoralis major muscular flap transfer: A prospective study of 16 patients IX. Zhang [et al.] // Oncology Letters. - 2015. - V. 10. -N.I.- P. 372-78.

147. Sammut L. Physical Activity and Quality of Life in Head and Neck Cancer Survivors: A Literature Review / L. Sammut, M. Ward, N. Patel / Intjof Sports Medicine. - 2014. - V. 35. -N.9. - P. 794-99.

148. Sandhir R. K. Learn to climb the simple reconstructive ladder properly for optimum results / R.K. Sandhir // Indian Journal of Plastic Surgery. Sandhir // Indian Journal of Plastic Surgery. - 2018. - V. 51. - N.3. - P. 331-32.

149. Seidenberg, B. The technique of anastomosing small arteries / B.

Seidenberg, E.S. Hurwitt, C. Carton // Surg Gynecol Obstet. - 1958. - V.106.-P. 743-6.

150. Shoulder morbidity after pectoralis major flap reconstruction / J. Refos [et al] // Head & Neck. - 2016. - V. 38. -N. 8.- P. 1221-28.

151. Status of radiotherapy resources in Africa: an International Atomic Energy Agency analysis / M. Abdel-Wahab [et al.]. // The Lancet Oncology. - 2013. - V. 14. - №4. - P. 168 - 75.

152. Stephenson K.A. Do Proton Pump Inhibitors Reduce the Incidence of Pharyngocutaneous Fistula following Total Laryngectomy: a prospective randomised controlled trial / K.A. Stephenson, J.J. Fagan // Head Neck. Fagan // Head Neck. - 2015. - V. 37. - N. 2. - P. 2559.

153. Strauch B., Vasconez L., Herman C.K., Lee B.T.. Grabb's Encyclopedia of Flaps. Head and Neck 4th Edition. Vol 1. 2009, 1215 p. ISBN07181774926.

154. Structured review of papers reporting specific functions in patients with cancer of the head and neck: 2006-2013 / S.N. Rogers [et al. Rogers [et al.] // Br J Oral Maxillofac Surg. - 2016. - V. 54. - N.6. - P. 45-51.

155. Suicide risk among cancer survivors: Head and neck versus other cancers IN. Osazuwa-Peters [et al.] // Cancer. - 2018. - V. 124. - P. 1-8.

156. Supraclavicular flap as a salvage procedure in reconstruction of head and neck complex defects / H. R. Alves [et al.] //J. Plastic, Reconstructive and Aesthetic Surgery. - 2019. - V. 72, №4.-P.9- 14.

157. Subjective and objective appearance of head and neck cancer patients following microsurgical reconstruction and associated quality of life - A cross-sectional study / K. Kansy [et al] // Journal of Cranio-Maxillofacial Surgery. - 2018. - V. 46. - N.8.- P. 1275-84.

158. Survival patterns in squamous cell carcinoma of the head and neck: pain as an independent prognostic factor for survival / C.C. Reyes-Gibby [et al.] // J Pain. - 2014. -V.15.-N. 10. - P. 1015-22.

159. The Birth of Plastic Surgery: The Story of Nasal Reconstruction from the Edwin Smith Papyrus to the Twenty-First Century. Plastic and Reconstructive Surgery 11. S. Whitaker / - 2007. - V. 120. - N. 1. - P. 327-36.

160. The course of health-related quality of life in head and neck cancer patients treated with chemoradiation: a prospective cohort study /

I.M. Verdonck-de Leeuw [et al.] Radiother Oncol. - 2014. - V. 110.-P. 422-28.

161. The economic burden of head and neck cancer: a systematic literature review *I* E. Wissinger [et al.] // Pharmacoeconomics. - 2014.-V.32.-P. 865-82.

162. The Laparoscopically Harvested Omental Free Flap: A Compelling Option for Craniofacial and Cranial Base Reconstruction *I*

246

P. Costantino [et al.] // Journal of Neurological Surgery Part B: Skull Base. - 2016. - V. 78. -N. 2.- P. 191-96.

163. The Pectoralis Major Myocutaneous Pedicled Flap Revisited IS. Asamura [et al.] // Surgical Science. -2013.-V. 4, № 9. - P. 380-84.

164. Treatment of Older Patients with Head and Neck Cancer: A Review IN. A. VanderWalde [et al.] *11* The Oncologist. - 2013. - V. 18. -N. 5.-P.568-78.

165. Well-being and quality of life among oral cancer patients - Psychological vulnerability and coping responses upon entering initial treatment *I* A. S. Bachmann [et al.] // Journal of Cranio- Maxillofacial Surgery. - 2018. - V. 46, № 9. - P. 1637-1644.

166. Wolff K.D. Perforator flaps: the next step in the reconstructive ladder? *I* K.D. Wolff // British Journal of Oral and Maxillofacial Surgery. - 2015. - V. 53. - N.9.- P. 787-95.

167. Wolff K.D. The diagnosis and treatment of oral cavity cancer *I* K.D. Wolff, M. Follmann, A. Nast *11* Deutsches Arzteblatt international. - 2012. - V. 109. - N. 48. - P. 829-35.

168. World Gastroenterology Organisation Global Guidelines *I* J.R. Malagelada [et al. Malagelada [et al.] // Journal of Clinical Gastroenterology. - 2015. - V. 49.-N.5.-P.370-78.

169. Worldwide Trends in Incidence Rates for Oral Cavity and Oropharyngeal Cancers *I* A.K. Chaturvedi [et al.] // J Clin Oncol. - 2013. - V. 31. - N. 36. - P. 4550-59.

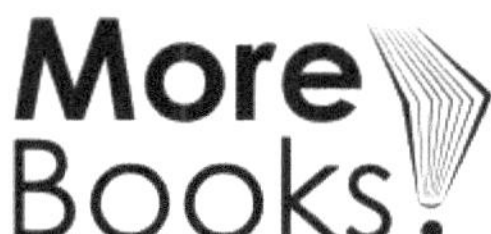

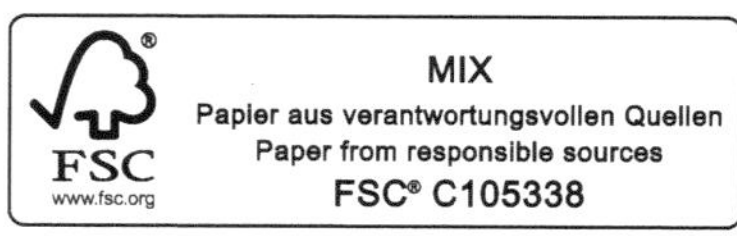

Printed by Books on Demand GmbH, Norderstedt / Germany